THE 7 SECRETS OF RAISING HAPPY EATERS

Why french kids eat everything
and how yours can too

KAREN LE BILLON

piatkus

PIATKUS

First published in the US as *Getting to Yum* in 2014 by William Morrow,
an imprint of HarperCollinsPublishers

First published in Great Britain in 2014 by Piatkus

Copyright © 2014 Karen Bakker Le Billon

The moral right of the author has been asserted.

A CIP catalogue record for this book
is available from the British Library.

ISBN 978-0-349-40444-8

Illustrations © Sarah Jane Wright

Typeset in Sabon by M Rules
Printed in Great Britain by Clays Ltd, St Ives plc

Papers used by Piatkus are from well-managed forests
and other responsible sources.

MIX
Paper from
responsible sources
FSC
www.fsc.org   FSC® C104740

To Sophie and Claire, my best "taste testers"

About the author

Karen Le Billon is a writer and teacher with a Ph.D from Oxford. The recipient of numerous awards, including a Rhodes Scholarship, Canada's Top 40 Under 40 award, and a national food writing award (Taste Canada), she is a Jamie Oliver Food Foundation's Real Food Advocate. Karen has published five scholarly books, as well as *French Kids Eat Everything*, the forerunner to this book. For many years she and her family have divided their time between Canada and France.

www.GettingToYum.com

Note: this book was published in the US and Canada as *Getting to Yum*. You'll find lots of additional information, including recipes and practical tips, on the Getting to Yum website.

Contents

Games and Experiments

Foreword

Obesity rates have skyrocketed in the past several decades, largely driven by unhealthful lifestyle behaviors in an increasingly automated "on the go" world. Aggressive food marketing has also fueled the childhood obesity epidemic by inducing children to crave high-calorie, low-nutrient foods and providing families with economic incentives to purchase them. Now more than ever, parents need effective strategies to help their children develop healthful eating habits for life.

As a pediatrician with expertise in pediatric obesity, one of the questions I am frequently asked is "How do we get children to eat what is good for them?" While this might seem like a simple question, the answer is incredibly complex. Karen Le Billon offered some thought-provoking ideas in her *New York Times* article "Why French Parents Are Superior (in One Way)." In it, Karen described how French parents effectively teach their children that "good-for-you foods" taste good, while American families often unwittingly do the opposite. In striking contrast to the limited repertoire of tastes preferred by many American children (and children in many other nations), the majority of French children learn to accept a large variety of tastes, flavors, and textures from an early age, and most of what they eat is healthy. It's not surprising then that North American children are three times more likely to be overweight than French children. Intrigued, I picked up a copy of Karen's first book, *French Kids Eat Everything*, and was transported to a small French town filled with wonderful flavors where Karen and her husband successfully converted their two children from picky eaters to foodie omnivores with the help of forward-thinking government-backed nutrition policies and savvy parenting strategies.

In her long-awaited second book, *The 7 Secrets of Raising Happy Eaters*, Karen translates the current scientific evidence and her own experience transforming her children's eating behaviors in France into a treasure trove of valuable lessons to help parents everywhere to do the same. Her "Secrets" offer carefully researched, evidence-based yet highly practical advice to help parents tame finicky eaters. Karen provides a great explanation of how children develop tastes and how this impacts their willingness to accept new foods. She then offers insightful and practical strategies to get children to try new foods through taste-training experiments that teach children (and their parents) important but often-neglected food experience skills in a non-threatening and fun way. I was particularly impressed to see that Karen adopts the avant-garde concept of *parents themselves* marketing healthy foods to children; the latest research has shown this to be a much more effective approach than sneaking foods into children's diets.

As a medical educator and the mother of four children with very distinct personalities and taste preferences, I am always looking for evidence-based, adaptable, and user-friendly materials I can use at home and with my families at work. My sometimes-finicky children and I have had a lot of fun trying some of the taste experiments in this book (they recently discovered they like/are okay with grapefruit), and my kids have declared several of our "test" recipes positively yummy!

The 7 Secrets of Raising Happy Eaters is a must-read for parents who want to not only teach but also show their children that healthful foods can truly be "yummy." This book beckons families to embark on a taste discovery adventure and methodically shows them that food can be a great source of joy and exploration. I thoroughly enjoyed the adventure with my family and hope that your family will enjoy it, too. Welcome aboard!

Dr. Jenny Cheng
Pediatrician and Clinical Director
One Step Ahead (Preventive Weight Management) Program
Harvard Medical School

Introduction

When I first met Jessica, her 3-year-old son Lucas would not eat a single vegetable. Not one! Among Lucas's list of forbidden foods were meat (with the exception of hot dogs), "mushy" foods (even roasted potatoes), and "anything green." Jessica was at her wits' end. "The dinner table feels like a battleground. I leave feeling so stressed. My husband and I don't know what else to do," she told me.

A few months after adopting the taste-training method in this book, Lucas's eating habits dramatically improved. Previously off-limits foods were now among Lucas's favorites: green beans, oranges, grapefruit—even raw spinach! Best of all, Lucas's baby sister, who benefited from taste training right from the start, happily eats anything put in front of her. "As a result of taste training," Jessica explained, "we've adopted new routines that have changed our family's eating habits for the better."

What is taste training, and why is it useful for parents?

Taste training is a hands-on, practical approach to food education that uses games and fun activities to help children learn to like healthy foods. The underlying principle is that children can *learn* to eat well, just as they learn to read. The idea that taste can be taught is a hopeful, positive message. The goal is simple: children will enjoy eating healthy foods because they *want* to (not because they *have* to). Your children will develop positive eating routines (*how, where,* and *when* to eat) that foster balanced appetites and healthy attitudes to food. They'll be healthy, happy, savvy eaters.

Of course, many food cultures—the French, the Italians, the Japanese, to name a few—have been practicing their version of taste training for generations. It's only recently that scientists and educators have studied the effects of taste training, and explained how and why it works so well. Researchers have spent the past few decades doing hundreds of amazing (and sometimes downright funny) experiments on babies and children: feeding babies slightly acidic water (their "sour face" looks just like an adult's); asking toddlers to eat fake green "grasshopper" icing (they will, happily); or dyeing food blue to see if peer pressure works to encourage reluctant kids to eat "scary" things (it does).

The core message of the scientific research on taste training is simple and inspiring: kids can actually learn to like new tastes (even if they are cautious about them at first). And that's not all. Specific taste-training techniques improve children's eating habits, make them more willing to try new foods, and change their long-term eating habits for the better. Kids who have gone through taste training eat healthy foods more regularly and eagerly, even months after the taste training is over.[1] In fact, scientific studies show that taste training works better than nutrition-focused education methods![2]

Our family's story: Curing picky eating

How do I know so much about children and food? My best qualification is being a mom to two wonderful daughters who were both picky eaters (one of those "blessed obstacles" that was a source of enormous stress when I was a new mother). I'm also a university professor, so I love digging for answers to complex problems. These two parts of my identity collided when my husband and I moved to France with our two young daughters, who were then subsisting on a "beige food" diet (pasta,

Cheerios, buttered toast, and crackers—you get the idea!). Because taste training is widespread in French homes and schools, my daughters received a food education similar to what I describe in this book. Within a year, the two girls (then 5 and 2) were eating—and loving—a huge range of foods, including beet salad, creamed spinach, broccoli, and mussels. (No, I am not making this up!)

I was so inspired by the positive change in our family's eating habits—and convinced that we had learned life-changing lessons that could be of use to parents worldwide—that I wrote a book about our experience, *French Kids Eat Everything*, which has gone on to be published in a dozen countries and ten languages. Readers wrote to me with heartfelt stories about how the ideas in *French Kids* inspired them to feed their families better. Others requested more recipes, tips, and practical advice. "The memoir was a great read," wrote one mom, "but when are you coming out with *the* parenting book we're all looking for?" So I've spent the past two years exploring and integrating research from many different fields: education, medicine, neurobiology, nutrition, psychology, sociology, and even comparative anthropology. In *The 7 Secrets of Raising Happy Eaters*, I've distilled the results down into key lessons and strategies for parents. (And I let off steam in the kitchen by developing and testing the recipes on my own family!)

I've been blessed to share the journey of writing this book with more than two dozen test families as well as more than 40 preschoolers at the Alphabet Academy in Connecticut. Their amazing stories and breakthroughs appear throughout this book and will, I hope, inspire you as much as they did me.

Could *my* family benefit from taste training?

Have you ever found yourself thinking any of these things:

- I know *what* my child should be eating, but I can't figure out *how* to get them to eat it!

- I want my child to eat better, but I don't want to use force, bribery, nagging, or begging.
- I often struggle to get my child to eat the recommended five servings of fruits and vegetables per day.
- My child reacts strongly or even refuses to eat when I serve new foods.
- I frequently make two or more meals at mealtime— one for the adults and one for each child.
- I sometimes substitute "kids' food" for healthier foods that my child rejects.
- Feeding my child is a source of stress.

If you responded "yes" to any of these statements, then this book is for you.

How does taste training work?

Taste training has a simple goal: to help you teach your child to *enjoy* being a healthy eater. Because we often assume that kids' tastes are innate, teaching a child to eat might sound odd. How often have you heard a parent say, "My kid is such a picky eater!"? We don't often think of eating as something that we *learn*; rather, we assume that eating is just something that we *do*. But kids *can* learn—and be taught—to eat well.

In order to achieve this goal, taste training involves three basic activities—fun games, simple recipes, and healthy eating routines—introduced in a strategic sequence: the "Seven Secrets" of healthy eating for kids. The underlying principle is that by improving *how, when*, and *why* you eat, you can improve *what* you eat.

Secret 1 explains how to *teach* your kids to enjoy tasting new foods. Secret 2 reveals how to use the power of food marketing to make healthy food more appealing for kids. Secret 3 helps you overhaul your family's eating routine through eliminating random snacking. Secret 4 introduces some mealtime magic: rituals and routines that make kids—and adults—eager to come to the table (and happy to stay there for a full meal). Secret 5 explains how to wean your kids off "kids' food" (if that's what they're used to eating). Most kids will feel more enthusiastic about this if they're helping in the kitchen—which is why Secret 6 is about child-led participation in cooking and family meal planning. And because parental emotions and attitudes are a key ingredient in your success, Secret 7 reveals techniques for keeping a Zen attitude despite the angst often associated with feeding our kids.

How do the games help?

Each of the Seven Secrets is associated with a set of fun games and experiments. Games are a fun, light-hearted yet effective way to introduce your child to new ways of eating and to deepen their understanding of food. The taste-training games (some of which are actually basic science experiments) are based on principles of experiential education. The underlying idea is simple (and backed up by research): kids need to *experience* what they are learning, in a "hands-on" way, not simply be told what to do.[3] Plus, games make learning to like new foods fun—for kids and adults alike.

Some of the games help children understand how eating relates to all five senses (touch, smell, sight, hearing, taste). As children become more comfortable with the physical sensations that different foods evoke, they become more confident eaters.[4] For example, Game 9 (The Sour Fruit Game) on page 83 teaches children that a grapefruit tastes *sour*, but that this taste is *not unpleasant*. Many of my test families' children became grapefruit lovers after playing this game!

Other games are designed to solve (or prevent) common childhood eating issues, as shown in the list that follows. For example, children who have difficulty mixing foods of different textures may find Game 16 (The Mixing Game) to be helpful.

How the Games Can Help

If your child has difficulty with this ...	Try this!
Eating different foods mixed together	Game 16: The Mixing Game (page 144)
Accepting the texture of specific foods	Game 13: Terrific Textures (page 123)
Eating too quickly	Game 18: The Slow Food Experiment (page 161)
Disliking sour foods	Game 9: The Sour Fruit Game (page 83)
Accepting changes to their favorite dishes	Game 19: The Same Food Three Ways Experiment (page 162)
Being sensitive to strong tastes	Game 3: Tasty Taste Buds (page 42)
	Game 4: The Supertaster Game (page 44)
Refusing to eat healthy foods	Game 5: The Silly Name Game (page 64)
Preferring junk food to healthy food	Game 6: The Smell–Taste Experiment (page 65)
	Game 8: Store Brand versus Name Brand Blind Taste Test (page 68)
	Game 14: The Color Confusion Experiment (page 127)
	Game 15: The Yogurt Game (page 128)
Sitting still at the table	Game 12: The Rose, Thorn, and Bud Game (page 105)
Eating salad	Game 17: Make-Your-Own Kids' Salad Game (page 146)

How do the recipes work with the taste-training approach?

The recipes in this book are designed in a sequence, with age-appropriate recipes for babies (approximately 9 to 18 months), toddlers (18 months to 4 years), preschoolers (4 to 6 years), and school-age children (6 years and older). The idea is simple: just as you teach a child math in a series of small steps, so too do you teach a child to eat in a series of steps. You start by exposing babies to basic tastes (as you would teach them to count to 10). Then, you add textures, particularly at the toddler stage (as you would teach them to count even higher and introduce number sequences). Preschoolers then begin expanding their range of knowledge about food as they try new taste/texture combinations (addition and subtraction). Finally, they're able to eat like adults (advanced calculus—kidding!). The recipes are designed to follow this sequence, and progressively introduce more complex tastes and textures to your child's diet. Take red peppers, for example: the recipes include a Roasted Red Pepper and Tomato Soup (page 254) for babies, followed by Red Rocket Hummus (page 255) for toddlers, Pinwheel Pepper Wraps (page 257) for preschoolers, and Ratatouille (page 258) for older kids. The beauty of this approach is that each of these recipes is designed to be tasty for adults, too—even the purée, which is actually a simple soup.

The recipes are also designed to be deliberately adventurous. You might be surprised by some of the ingredients (such as sage or anchovies), but please put your doubts aside. You may find (as my test families often did) that your kids can enjoy these ingredients, even if they aren't usually considered typical kids' food.

Is taste training like sleep training?

Eating is a basic bodily function, like sleeping. But eating *well* is a complex skill that takes years to acquire. Taste training is best compared with reading. Learning to read well takes time and effort; it takes years before a child becomes a competent, confident reader. But this doesn't mean that reading is unpleasant. And neither is taste training. Curling up with a young child and reading them a book is one of the cosiest things you could imagine. Remember how excited you were to rediscover your favorite kids' books with your child? Or what it was like when your child learned to walk or managed to bicycle on their own for the very first time? Now imagine you felt that way about teaching them about eating, about exploring the wonderful world of food together. What if you felt that way about introducing new foods—as something to be anticipated and celebrated?

Can *all* children learn to eat well?

Your belief in your child's capacity to become a competent eater is a key factor in their success. Some children will take longer (and some *much* longer) than others, but most children *can* learn to eat well. However, if you suspect your child has particular difficulty eating, they may have an underlying medical issue (including allergies, autism spectrum disorder, or a sensory processing disorder) that is best dealt with in consultation with your health-care provider.

At what age can I start taste training?

Taste training can be started at any age. (In fact, some of my test families reported their biggest successes with formerly picky *parents*!) Although it is easier with younger children, it's never too late to start. If your children are older (as mine were when I started), don't worry: it may take a little longer, but kids are remarkably adaptable. For older kids, *The 7 Secrets of Raising Happy Eaters* can work as a "rehab" program, helping your children to wean themselves from processed foods and create new, positive eating habits. If you have a baby under the age of 2, your journey will be much easier. Taste training at this age is like preventive medicine. Your goal will be to nip picky eating in the bud and perhaps even prevent it from appearing altogether. Plus, you'll be able to take full advantage of the simple recipes at the back of this book. If you're starting at this age, you're lucky! You can create healthy eating routines right from the start.

Won't kids just grow out of picky eating on their own?

The majority of children (around 3 out of 4 in most studies) are selective about the foods they eat: rejecting new foods, preferring a small range of favorite foods, and even developing deep attachments to specific "fetish" foods (such as pasta). Pickiness, in other words, is normal for some children. But with simple taste-training techniques even the most hard-core picky eaters will diversify their diets.

At this point you may be congratulating yourself, saying, "My child isn't picky!" Good for you (and for them)—but don't celebrate too soon. Selective eating varies with age, in a fairly predictable pattern. It often appears during toddlerhood, but can also occur at other ages, for different reasons. About 4 out of 10 babies are eager eaters (particularly when they're hungry) who will enjoy or at least try new foods. Another 4 out of those 10 babies are strong-willed eaters who show strong food preferences right from the start. About 2 in 10 will be fussy eaters right from the start.

From about the age of 2 and up, some previously eager or strong-willed eaters will start to be selective. They might be fussy (refusing foods they've previously eaten and enjoyed, and often changing preferences from one day to the next) and/or picky (refusing to try new foods and making demands to eat familiar foods). Picky eating (termed "neophobia," or the fear of new foods) often emerges at around the age of 2 and usually peaks at about 4 or 5. Some research suggests that boys, on average, tend to be pickier than girls at this age.[5]

By the time they start school, most children have a consistent sense of their likes and dislikes, and these preferences tend to remain stable over time. By the ages of 10 to 12, picky eating declines in most children, although food preferences change as children approach adolescence. If the family is experiencing power struggles over food, or an adolescent is experiencing other personal issues, pickiness may intensify. Pickiness may be related, for example, to concerns over personal health, body image, or eating disorders. Eventually, however, most children grow out of picky eating.

When this pattern of development was first explained to me, I was relieved. I realized that picky eating was a normal phase of development for many kids that arises from a combination of factors, including a child's innate eating type, family food habits and routines, and social pressures and experiences inside and outside the home. No more guilt! (Getting rid of guilt is one of the first steps in developing a healthy family eating routine.)

Most important, I also realized there was something I—and all parents—could do about picky eating. For most kids, picky eating is a phase, not a lifelong condition. Just as firm, responsive parenting can help kids grow out of the "no" phase, taste training can help your child grow out of picky eating.

What if my child resists? Won't it make picky eating worse?

If you're worried about resistance, start with the games listed in each chapter. They're great for awakening your child's natural curiosity about food. They'll help you teach your child to like the taste of healthy foods and to adopt healthy eating habits throughout the day. The premise of this approach is that food is fun.

Yes, that's right. *Food is fun.* What does this mean? It means that you *can* enjoy meals with your children. You may not believe it right at this moment (and, believe me, when struggling with my young children's eating habits, I wouldn't have believed it either), but you and your child *can* have fun trying healthy new foods.

For really resistant kids, you might want to skip ahead to Secrets 6 and 7. Secret 6 explains how to replace pressure with kids' participation and introduces "child-led" learning strategies that are designed to get your child working with you rather than against you. Secret 7 has some suggestions for maintaining parental calm and detachment in stressful eating situations: the more relaxed (yet firm) you are when providing guidance, the more successful you are likely to be.

What about allergies?

Taste training is based on the belief that we don't need to be afraid of introducing a wide variety of foods and tastes to children of all ages (in fact, the younger the better). This approach is supported by recent medical advice that encourages parents not to delay the introduction of *any* foods—even those previously thought of as "allergenic"—to babies older than 6 months. In fact, doctors are now studying the possibility that delaying the introduction of allergenic foods—such as peanuts—may *increase* the chance of developing allergies. This idea (not yet scientifically proven) suggests that eating a wide variety of foods may actually protect against allergies. In summary, doctors recommend that a wide variety of foods be introduced early and eaten regularly.[6] Taste training offers a method that enables you to put this advice into practice.

What taste training is not

Taste training is *not* a method for producing "perfect" eaters (there is no such thing!). Nor does it assume that your child will eat everything. Children, just like adults, have taste preferences that should be respected.

Taste training is not about nutritional education. Extensive research shows that nutritional education is not very helpful for *changing* behavior or creating positive behaviors. In other words, getting your child to eat well has very little to do with nutrition. Don't get me wrong, nutrition is important—micronutrient deficiencies (particularly iron, zinc, and calcium) are still an issue for too many children, even in relatively wealthy societies—but research has shown time and again that using nutrition-based arguments is not the best way to convince your child to eat better.

Taste training is not a "blame and shame" approach to eating. Rather, it's a positive approach that treats food as a source of joy and exploration, like a shared adventure. It's about *how* we might inspire our children—and ourselves—to eat better, because it's something that they—and we—*enjoy* doing. So you won't hear me repeating the well-known information about the problems. Instead, we'll focus on solutions.

Finally, taste training is not about dieting or eating only "healthy" food (however that is defined). The recipes provided in the second part of the book focus on fruits and vegetables, which tend to be what children have a harder time learning to like. But I like to steer clear of labels (like "good" and "bad" foods). Rather, you'll teach your child that there are different approaches to foods: some they can eat regularly and some are occasional treats. My view is that there is nothing wrong with treats—in moderation. In fact, "moderation rather than deprivation" is a key principle of this approach. Research shows that depriving children of certain foods makes them more likely to crave them. Equally, forcing children to eat "healthy" foods (or using treats as a bribe) makes it more probable that children will dislike those foods. Taste training takes a different approach: assuming that children can and will like all sorts of foods because they are inherently tasty. Broccoli . . . *yum!* That's why snack and dessert recipes are included, too.

How long will this take?

You may be thinking, *Sounds good, but how quickly will I see a change?* I won't kid you: it's not an instant process. Good eating doesn't happen overnight. If you're firm about the new approaches that you adopt, you will see changes in most toddlers within a week or two. School-age children will take longer. Adolescents might take up to a month or more. Be patient and gently persistent.

How much time per week will this take? If you play one game every day and introduce one new recipe a week, then you'll be spending 30 minutes a week on taste training—that's less than 5 minutes per day! Be warned, however: taste training grows on you. As my test families found out, once you start—and once your child surprises you with their breakthrough new food "likes"—you won't want to stop. Most test families found themselves doing more, not less, taste training over time.

Your family food journey is likely to be a bit of a rollercoaster ride. Your child will nibble on broccoli one day and balk at it the next. They'll whine at the table and forget their manners, then surprise you with their sweetness. Some family meals will be grumpy—this is where mindful eating can help. When applied to parents, I take it to mean "Take a deep breath, resist the temptation to yell or scold, and remember that this too shall pass." Remember that taste training, in the long run, will be worth it. You'll be spending less time in the kitchen because you'll be introducing the principle of "one family, one meal" to your household and eliminating short-order cooking. Your child will be less fussy at mealtimes and, in most cases, will have become an "easy eater." Ultimately, you'll be able to focus more on enjoying your child rather than being stressed about what they do (or don't) eat—and shouldn't that be the ultimate goal?

Let your family food adventure begin!

Love,

Karen

P.S. I've included lots of helpful information on my website **GettingToYum.com,** including recipes, menus, research sources, tips, and more. Please do visit!

The 7 Secrets of Raising Eager Eaters

Secret 1

Kids Can *Learn* to Love Healthy Foods: Here's How to Teach Them

Imagine that one day you travel to another country, somewhere far away, somewhere quite different. Soon after arriving, you meet a family with young children. Curious, the parents ask you to explain what children "back home" typically like to eat. What comes to mind? If you've been raised in North America, you probably think of hot dogs, pizza, and soda. Or you may think of baby food: white rice cereal or maybe applesauce. Stereotypical kids' food.

Now imagine what happens when you ask that family what *their* kids eat. Depending on where you are, you'll get very different answers. In India, little kids eat curries (albeit milder versions than the adult variety); young children encounter herbs and spices like mint, turmeric, and cinnamon early on. Mexican toddlers begin eating hot sauce before they start first grade. In Korea, even young kids love sour kimchi (a pickled cabbage and vegetable dish), and a school lunch might include seaweed or bean sprout soup, pickled radish, or octopus stir-fry. In Japan, when not nibbling on *natto* (fermented soybeans), young children are served rice porridge topped with chopped tofu, fish (fresh or dried), or vegetables. In Italy, babies' cereals are mixed with *brodo* (a delicious vegetable stock seasoned with garlic and topped with Parmesan and olive oil). Jarred Italian baby food options include rabbit and even horsemeat. I've seen Italian mothers spoon-feeding café latté (presumably single-shot!) to their stroller-bound babies, both mom and tot cooing happily all the while. Seaweed and seal blubber (rich in vitamin C) are traditional first foods for Inuit babies, followed by whale meat and bush foods (such as caribou meat). In France, recommended first foods for babies include leek soup and endive. One of the top-selling French baby cookbooks includes vegetables such as artichoke, celery, and cauliflower for babies, and features dishes like sea bass with fennel ("why not serve it for your child's first birthday meal?"). For the adventurous toddler, the same cookbook features "scallop tartare" (yes, raw seafood!) topped with minced pickles, capers, and white pepper.

These examples might seem strange at first, but they're actually not. All over the world, parents introduce young children to the varied flavors of their particular food culture. That means introducing them to spicy foods, sour foods, salty foods, sweet foods—strong tastes of all kinds, even the ones that current North American culture would say kids "can't" like.

Your grandparents would probably have been perplexed by the idea of "kids' food"; when they were young, kids ate the same food as everyone else. This is, of course, partly practical: without refrigeration, and with seasonal (and often limited) food choices, people cooked what they had and ate because they were hungry. Parents had no reason to believe that their kids wouldn't like the food that they ate. Industrial food culture has turned this relationship on its head. We now assume that kids prefer "kids' food," so that's (by and large) what we feed them.

But what if we took a more positive approach and assumed the opposite: that kids can actually *enjoy* eating a wide variety of foods? Why wouldn't we want children to enjoy the subtle flavor of, say, broccoli? If parents believe these vegetables are tasty and eat them themselves, their child will eventually learn to eat a healthy, diverse diet. And if a child is timid about a new vegetable and says "I hate it," a parent could (and should) help them figure out ways to like the new vegetable. As described in the experiment that follows, the starting point is your expectations of your child, which help set them up for success (or failure).

The Pygmalion effect

How important are our beliefs about our children's capacity to learn? Very important, as Harvard researcher Robert Rosenthal found out. In 1965, Rosenthal (a psychologist) and Lenore Jacobsen (an elementary school principal) conducted an unorthodox experiment in a California public school. They told teachers that they had used a Harvard-designed test (the Harvard Test of Inflected Acquisition) to identify which students were about to go through an intellectual growth spurt. The teachers were excited, as the Harvard method was supposed to help them target and support kids' learning. But here's the thing about Rosenthal's experiment: it was based on a lie. The Test of Inflected Acquisition didn't exist. And the students identified as being about to "spurt" intellectually were chosen at random.[1]

Rosenthal hoped to prove that teachers' expectations of students influenced how well students actually performed. He was proven right. When his team came back to the school several months later, the selected children had significantly improved their school performance. Even Rosenthal was surprised by how much the children had improved; he'd expected a small difference, but some children had gone from being C students to A students. He was also astounded by another result: the children had also gained in IQ, up to 40 points higher than the students who were not selected!

His conclusion? Teachers' expectations of how much children *could* learn powerfully influenced how much they *actually* learned. Rosenthal called this the "Pygmalion Effect," based on the famous play by George Bernard Shaw (and later the movie *My Fair Lady*) in which working-class Eliza Doolittle is taught by Professor Henry Higgins to lose her Cockney accent and adopt the manners of a lady, confounding the audience's beliefs about the natural inferiority of the "lower" classes.

Rosenthal's experiment had an enormous social impact because it proved that adults' expectations of children have an enormous influence on how children actually behave and learn—and the effect is most pronounced in young children. Perhaps most important, the experiment demonstrates the power of labels. If you label your son a picky eater, he will likely become one. If you tell your daughter there are some foods she doesn't like, she'll probably believe you. If you yourself believe that some foods (such as vegetables) are not tasty, your kids will probably feel the same way.

This notion of labels really hit home with my friend Kate, who only recently realized that her father didn't like broccoli yet dutifully ate it for 20 years. His devotion paid off: although he still doesn't like broccoli, it's Kate and her sister Lauren's favorite vegetable! The simple message: if you want your kids to eat something, eat it in front of them with obvious enjoyment. And tell them it's tasty.

The opposite is also true: if you act alarmed when your 3-year-old reaches for a piece of grapefruit (as one dad did when visiting our house for brunch) and say "Ooh, that's too acidic for you" in an alarmed voice (which is what he did), your toddler will probably recoil and decide she doesn't like it (which is exactly what his child did). Kids naturally feel wary of foods that their parents dislike. This behavior is, of course, a useful protective mechanism, but it can be taken too far. When your child encounters a new food, try simply encouraging them to try it— with curiosity and without judgment.

Kids are "emerging eaters"

Instead of labeling your child a picky eater, try thinking of them as a "learning" or "emerging" eater. Your child will believe that it's normal to learn to like new foods, and they'll naturally turn to you to help them to do so. If you avoid telling them (either directly or indirectly) that there are good- or bad-tasting foods, and rather describe food as having *interesting* tastes, they might surprise you with their interest in new foods.

Here's a simple example from our family. A few years ago we were at our local neighborhood block party in Vancouver, a city lucky enough to be home to a diverse set of cuisines. One of the treats on offer was a spicy snack: wasabi-flavored seaweed (wasabi—also known as Japanese horseradish—is a pale green paste with a hot mustard taste). Our neighbor offered me some, and then my 4-year-old daughter, Claire, asked for a piece. "Ooh, she'll find that too spicy, I think!" my neighbor replied as she angled the tray away from Claire. But Claire asked again, and I handed her half of my piece. As our neighbor backed up and waited for the (she thought) inevitable wail, I told Claire, "Try it—you'll like it! It's really tasty!" As Claire happily munched on her piece and asked for my other half, our per-plexed neighbor tried one more time: "It's super-spicy, isn't it?" Claire nodded, while blithely savoring the snack and even asking for another piece.

This wasn't an isolated incident. Before the age of 5, Claire was also eating (and, more important, enjoying) Thai curries and tofu, sushi and spinach, broccoli and beets, Roquefort cheese, and more. This doesn't mean that she eats everything—she has a serious scrambled egg hang-up, for some reason—but she does eat most things. She and her older sister, Sophie (now 9), weren't born liking these foods, of course. They *learned* to enjoy eating them. In fact, young kids are open to eating a much broader range of foods than we think.

There's a comb in my milk ... *yum!*

Intrigued by young children's attitudes toward food, Paul Rozin (a psychologist at the University of Pennsylvania) decided to study how humans develop feelings of disgust. His experiments were simple. In one case, children listened to a story in which a contaminant (a grasshopper, a leaf, and even "doggie doo") falls into a glass of milk. After each sentence, children were asked how much they would like to drink the milk, rating their responses with a smiley face chart. Another experiment asked children to consume foods that seemed to be contaminated; for example, the experimenter pretended to comb their hair, then dipped the comb in a glass of juice, removed it, and asked the child to drink the juice.[2] Over the years, the experimenters tried many different strategies, including my favorite: asking toddlers to eat short-bread sprinkled with "grasshopper powder" (flour, sugar, green food coloring). The adults who participated in the experiment were exposed to additional scenarios, which included stirring soup with a never-used comb or fly swatter.

How did the kids and adults react to Rozin's experiments? Older kids wouldn't even dream of accepting the drink or soup until the glass was washed—and even then, half of them still refused. The adults were the most resistant: many not only refused to taste, but suggested the now-contaminated glass or bowl should simply be thrown out. However, the youngest children (3-year-olds) were happy to sip their milk, slurp their juice, and chomp their grasshopper powder-topped cookies. They didn't appear to distinguish between foods that were dangerous, disgusting, or simply inappropriate.

As Rozin summed it up: "Young children seem to believe that things that are bad for them will taste bad. And things that are good for them will taste good." So how does a child learn that broccoli is good *and* tastes good, too? Not on their own, Rozin's research suggests. Rather, children learn food *dislikes* from the adults and other kids around them. And as every parent knows, food preferences are hard to change once they're established.[3]

Supertasters

Kids are not a blank slate, however. Recent discoveries have shown that taste sensitivity is, to some extent, genetic. University of Florida researcher Linda Bartoshuk studies the genetic variations in taste perception and categorizes people three ways: supertasters, average tasters, and non-tasters.[4]

For supertasters, about 25 percent of the American population, bitter foods taste much more bitter and sweeter foods much more sweet.[5] "Average tasters" make up 50 percent of the population. The remaining 25 percent are the "non-tasters," who are much less sensitive to any taste sensation. As Bartoshuk explains, "Supertasters live in a 'neon' world of taste, while non-tasters are in a 'pastel' world."[6] I think I have one child on each extreme of the spectrum: my older daughter will gasp in pain and immediately spit out any raw garlic that accidentally finds its way into her food. My younger daughter will, on the other hand, chew on it thoughtfully, without much obvious discomfort. This doesn't mean that my older daughter doesn't enjoy strong flavors (she loves Thai curry, for example), but it does take her a little longer to learn to like them.

Why are kids so different from one another? Part of the reason may be physiological: they may have a different density of fungiform papillae (taste buds). Each taste bud is associated with a bundle of nerves that sends pain signals to the brain. More taste buds translate into a stronger pain sensation, and more sensitive taste perception in general.[7] (Interestingly, women are more likely to be supertasters because they tend to have more taste buds than men.[8])

The important thing to remember is that children have (on average) more taste buds than adults. In other words, most children will have a more sensitive sense of taste than most adults. This is why lots of practice—through repeated tasting of new foods—is so important: *most* kids are likely to take longer than the average adult to get used to the new tastes of foods. Patient, gentle persistence is key to taste training.

Don't be worried about "funny faces"

When serving new foods to your children, be aware that their facial expressions may be misleading. Scientists have found that children's facial expressions are a good indicator of food likes, but not of food dislikes.[9] No one is sure why kids make such faces, but their expression may be a hangover from the "gusto-facial reflex" that newborn babies display when given acidic or bitter tastes. Even though kids have a cautious look on their face, or even wrinkle up their noses, that doesn't mean they dislike the new food. Rely on what children say rather than how they look.

The gusto-facial reflex

What happens if you give an infant a sip of a sweet liquid? And then a sour liquid? It turns out that all infants show the same reactions: happy-looking faces for sweet tastes, and grimaces for sour (and bitter and salty) tastes. These reactions are so universal, and so easily discernible, that when researchers took photos of the babies' faces and showed them to uninformed adults, the adults were easily able to tell what the babies had tasted. The gusto-facial reflex appears in the first day of life in children all over the world. Scientists thus term it an innate (observed at birth) reflex, rather than an acquired (or learned) reflex. It likely evolved due to its protective qualities (breast milk is sweet, and many toxins and poisons taste bitter). Children gradually learn to like a variety of tastes, but their "funny food faces" (which could to some extent be inadvertent) may persist until adolescence!

Practice, practice, practice

When was the last time you learned to like a new food? For most of us, it was a while ago. Just like kids, we get stuck in food habits. We've forgotten that we actually had to learn to like the foods we now enjoy (it took me years to enjoy the taste of coffee, for example). The good news is that kids (and adults, too) can learn to like new foods through repeated exposure: basically, practice makes perfect.[10]

Of course, you can overdo practicing. This is particularly the case for younger children (up until about the age of 7 or 8), for whom trying new foods is sometimes a big challenge. Introducing too many new foods to younger kids all at once might backfire, as they need a slower pace. It's about finding a balance: some variety and new foods, but not too much.[11] Once per day may work for many kids, but once per week might be better for others. You know your child best.

Just a little regular practice can bring results very quickly; having your child spend only 5 minutes per day trying new foods and practicing their habits quickly adds up. This is important because studies show that, on average, children need to taste a new food anywhere up to 12 times before they will happily eat it.[12] For example, 4-year-old Rena (one of my test family kids) wasn't so sure about cauliflower the first two times it was served. But the third time her mom served the Cauliflower Gratin recipe on page 232, both Rena and her little sister ate it without complaint (and even asked for more!).

Jon (from another test family) had a similar experience with his 13-year-old son, Michael, a confirmed picky eater. Described by his dad as "a kid who had probably never tried a green bean," Michael tried (with some reluctance) Green Beans Amandine (page 241). The first time he didn't finish his serving or express interest in having any more. The next week, however, Michael surprised his entire family by asking, "Why can't we have green beans more often?" Jon wrote to me afterward:

> *My wife and I were speechless. Now my son is asking for green beans! Remarkable. Illustrates how we let our misconceived assumptions about what children like and don't like get in the way of actually helping our kids to learn to like food.*

As both Michael and Rena's examples show, repeated *low-pressure* exposure to new food is critical to successful taste training. That's why I recommend that your family adopt this simple—but extremely effective—Family Food Rule:

You don't have to like it, but you do have to taste it.

Some readers will recognize this as one of the Food Rules I described in *French Kids Eat Everything,* written after our family spent a year in France. There, we saw the impressive (seemingly magical) results of asking children to taste everything prepared for them, even if they don't eat it. The more familiar something is, the more children tend to like it.[13] Your goal is to build that familiarity through regular repetition. Note: looking at the food isn't enough—children have to taste it (remember, it may take up to a dozen "tastes" before your child will eat a new food). Cautious kids will benefit from other types of exposure first: seeing, touching, and talking about the new food.[14]

Children quickly learn this rule, and sometimes even encourage each other to follow it, as did Rena. Only a few days into the taste-testing process, Rena started asking her parents what she would be eating for dinner. Meals became something to look forward to, to be curious about. Rena was proud of being the "big kid," chanting "you don't have to like it, you just have to try it" to encourage her little sister, Rachel (2½), to follow suit. Rachel even surprised her parents by being the more eager eater, particularly when brightly colored foods were served.

Even young children can encourage one another to taste test new foods, as Alexandra, a reader, wrote to me:

I made a version of Ratatouille today with vegetables we grew in our garden. With spoon in hand, my 2½-year-old son sat at the lunch table staring at his bowl and not touching a bite. Then, between mouthfuls, my 4-year-old daughter simply said, "You don't have to like it, but you have to try it." And try it he did ... until his whole bowl was empty and he asked for more.

—Alexandra

Banish the bland

Learning to like new things is even more complicated if your child prefers a fairly bland diet. The problem with the bland food approach is that it teaches kids to avoid strong tastes— which is what characterizes most healthy food. When they grow older, we worry that they don't eat the recommended amount of vegetables and fruits per day. And we *should* worry: child obesity rates are rapidly rising around the world, affecting our children's mental and physical health, their school performance, even their IQ.

Dr. Jatinder Bhatia, a pediatrician and member of the American Academy of Pediatrics Committee on Nutrition, recommends feeding mild curries to babies.[15] Indian parents feed curry to their babies from a very early age. The result is that they develop their baby's love of curry taste *before* they arrive at the "no" stage at around age 2. The same reasoning applies to all sorts of cultures, including Japan, where parents feed fish (*shirasu*) to infants.

The lesson here is simple: if you focus on developing a baby's palate early on, they'll be less likely to be extremely picky later in life. This is one reason why parents from other cultures are often mystified upon learning that North Americans serve mostly bland food to their babies. When I explained the approach recommended in my American baby books to my French friend Laurence, she asked, puzzled, "Are you training them to *dislike* most foods?"

This doesn't mean you should serve a blazingly hot curry to your 3-year-old tonight. It's a gradual process. Being good at something doesn't happen overnight. If you've ever taught a child to ride a bicycle, swim, or play the piano, you know that it takes time. *Lots* of time. Patient persistence is a parent's best friend. You may be surprised, like Françoise:

I never had the confidence to push new dishes and vegetables. I backed down too fast. Now I am more confident to keep trying things they've said they didn't like for years. I've been surprised by what my kids like and don't like, and have discovered many things about each child's preferences (I thought I knew them!). My 3-year-old was, I thought, my easiest eater, but then I realized that she liked healthy things but not necessarily new things—totally different. I'm also surprised that they liked the most adventurous tastes (apple curry soup) but not the sweet things (berry yogurt). We ordered lamb at a restaurant the other day, and they were fighting over it! So their taste buds have definitely developed.

—Françoise

Do your kids (and yourself) a "friendly flavor" favor

Many kids don't like the taste of vegetables on the first try. Nature seems to have unfairly stacked the deck. The tastes that our kids seem to love are exactly the same as the ones we can't resist as adults: sugar above all, but also salt and fat. In fact, as the processed food industry has discovered, the right combination of sugar, salt, and fat can even result in addiction-like symptoms in both kids and adults.[16]

The power of innate taste preferences is evident right from birth: newborns love sugar.[17] A drop of a sweet taste on an infant's tongue will result in a smile and the relaxation of baby's muscles—so much so that doctors call this the "analgesic" (pain-reducing) effect of sugar, and have actually tested the use of sugar solutions as a means of reducing infant pain during medical procedures.[18] (I don't think I would have signed up my girls for this experiment, but I'm glad some brave parents did.) Conversely, a drop of a sour taste will result in a reflex response that any parent will recognize: that dreaded pursing of lips and furrowing of the brow.

The preference for sweet isn't limited to North American food culture. Children around the world tend to prefer sweet, salty, and fatty flavors, and to be less fond of the sour, bitter, alkaline flavors that characterize vegetables. (Scientists don't know why this is the case, but believe that it may be due to an innate aversion to potential toxins and poisons, which tend to be sour and bitter.) It's no surprise that children like those same vegetables much more if they are flavored with a little fat (a dollop of butter, a drizzle of olive oil) or naturally sweet foods (leek purée mixed with a little pear, for example).

As you're conducting taste experiments at home, keep in mind that some children may benefit from the "friendly flavor" tactic. Simply put: if you use flavors your child already enjoys, they will be more willing to try (and more likely to enjoy) new foods.[19] Scientists call this effect "flavor conditioning," and have done many experiments on why and how it works. In one experiment, researchers added white sugar to grapefruit and found that children increased their liking for not just grapefruit, but all sour foods as a result.[20] Interestingly, serving flavorful preparations of fruits and vegetables to kids increased their subsequent liking for the plain versions of the vegetables; kids will "graduate" from grapefruit with sugar to plain grapefruit (as mine have done).[21]

Many parents use "flavor conditioning" already (think ketchup). There are lots of flavors to try: my kids love "green ketchup" (*Pistou*, page 368), a yummy veggie pesto sauce. Classic Vinaigrette (page 365) is a great dip for all sorts of vegetables (or use a salad dressing that your children like). Or keep it simple: butter or olive oil, with a pinch of salt, works wonders with most vegetables. Whatever condiments you choose (hummus, sweet-and-sour sauce, yogurt dip, or even ketchup) are fine; just be sure to expose your child to more than one "friendly flavor." Resist the temptation to coat everything in tomato ketchup![22] You want to program your child to prefer the taste of real food and to expect variety—not to get stuck liking just a few things. The more you can vary these flavors, the better.

Using the friendly flavor approach is a great way to gradually taste train your kids: you can use familiar flavors as building blocks to introduce more complex dishes to your child's repertoire. For example, our friend Laurence, who lives in the south of France, started off serving simple zucchini purée to her baby Antoine, then added parsley and tomatoes a few months later. By the time baby Antoine was 1½ years old, eggplant and peppers had been added, the texture had gone from smooth to lumpy, and Antoine was eating something that closely resembled the classic French stew ratatouille (see page 258).

How to teach a child to learn to like new foods

What would you do if a child was timid on the first day at a new school and said "I hate school"? You'd help them figure out ways to like school. You'd gently persist. Learning to like new foods—often one at a time—is similar.

How do you introduce new foods in a way that respects children's individual sensitivities? And how do you do this without force (which almost inevitably backfires)? One of the best ways is the taste test approach, in which you ask a child to taste a small amount but don't require them to eat it. When a child says "I don't like that food," they often mean "I don't know it." Being exposed to a new food in multiple ways helps children to tame their fears.

> *When we started taste testing and thinking about food like a mini-experiment, I began asking my kids questions when they didn't like a particular recipe. What don't you like: the texture, the smell, the appearance, or the other ingredients? This encouraged my kids to explore the depth of food and food combinations. Through this process, we discovered Kelly actually did like soup, but didn't enjoy the texture of celery, which was a huge breakthrough for her (the one person who didn't like soup in our soup-o-phile home). It was also through this process that I confirmed that my daughters found dressing to be too spicy, and lettuce too hard to get on a fork. That led me to rework the way I prepare salad, which they now love!*
> *—Lori*

A word of warning: avoid trying new foods if your child is feeling ill or if you're about to go on a long car ride and you know your child has a tendency to get carsick. Psychologists have found that humans are hard-wired to develop aversions to food they associate with illness. If you feed a person a new food and then make them feel ill shortly after, they'll develop an aversion for the odor and flavor of that food—even if it wasn't the cause of their illness.[23] But don't worry: if your child does develop a food aversion in this way, it probably won't last forever.

Ready, set ... taste!

So how do you put the ideas in this chapter into action? First, you can teach your child how to learn to like new foods using the step-by-step taste-testing method that follows. Once they've gotten used to taste testing, you can introduce new foods using the easy-to-make recipes in the second part of this book. You can also try following the family taste-testing plan on page 38. Follow this up with the four games starting on page 39 to introduce your child to some basic ideas about flavors and taste buds that will encourage them to broaden their palates. (Feel free to change the order of any of these steps to suit your family; for picky eaters you may want to start with the games.)

Taste Testing: A Step-by-Step Approach

1. **Pick a new food similar to something your child already likes.** If they like cucumbers, try thin slices of green pepper. If they like carrots, try red peppers. If they like one kind of bread, try a different kind of bread.
2. **Introduce it before you serve it.** Sounds silly, but this step is important because children are often wary of foods they don't recognize. For example, show your child a red pepper (the sweet, not spicy kind!). Go shopping with them and let them choose one to take home. Let them touch it and smell it. Cut it open and let them look at the intense color. Next, try a variety of ways to introduce red peppers to your family. Children may appreciate helping with cooking and serving "their" chosen vegetable. This will also help them make the connection between foods in different

forms—that raw tomato they're wary about tasting is the main ingredient in the pizza sauce they love. Introducing children to raw vegetables often helps them overcome their wariness of eating vegetables in cooked form.

3. **Serve a small amount, prepared as plainly as possible, but still packed with flavor.** Use a little tasting bowl or ramekin, or serve a taste on a small spoon. A little bit of carrot soup on a spoon looks a lot less intimidating than a huge bowl of soup on the table. For cautious kids, you can try putting a small dollop or dab of the new food on one of their favorite crackers (or simply bread, if they prefer that). Some children will be reassured if they're allowed to dab the food on the cracker themselves.

4. **Taste it yourself—and enjoy it!** Research shows that kids are more likely to be willing to try (and actually eat) a food if parents or peers try it first—and visibly enjoy it. (Don't fake it—they'll have you figured out in a flash.)

5. **Don't ask them to eat it; simply ask them to taste it.** The key is not to create stress around accepting or rejecting new foods. Simply ask the child to taste and get acquainted with the dish. Removing the pressure to eat (by asking them to just taste) means that they aren't resisting—they're just experimenting, in a low-pressure and encouraging environment. Try telling them, "Don't let the eyes do the work of the tongue." Kids judge foods primarily by appearance (color and texture).[24] This means they're more likely to be wary of new things. If you sprinkle chopped fresh parsley on their favorite pasta, their suspicions will be raised, even if it tastes pretty much the same. Encourage them to move beyond first impressions and actually taste things rather than pre-judge them. You might also want to tell reluctant children that they're

allowed to spit the food out (as politely as possible) or to simply test it with their tongue. In other words, they don't have to swallow the food that they're taste testing. Most important, try not to react negatively if your child decides not to eat the new food. A cheerful, firm comment ("You'll like it more the next time") sends the right message.

6. **Ask your child to talk about it.** Whatever you do, don't ask your child if they like the new food—you'll be setting yourself up for a "No!" Rather, ask them to describe the food in positive (or at least neutral) terms. If kids get used to saying "yuck" about anything unfamiliar, they'll risk getting stuck in a food-refusal rut. Describing the foods will help make the food more familiar. Ask your child to tell you what they think about the actual taste of the food, commenting on the flavors and textures they're encountering. Think of fun words you can teach your child to describe the different attributes of the food they are tasting: temperature (icy, lukewarm, steaming, scalding), taste (bitter, acidic, honeyed, savory, spicy, sweet-and-sour, tangy, zesty), texture (creamy, crunchy, crispy, crumbly, dry, fatty, fizzy, flaky, silky, tender, tough). Have fun thinking of new words or even inventing them—my younger daughter Claire likes to describe desserts she loves as "plummy"! By giving your child the language to describe their food, you'll find out what they like (as well as what they don't like) and be able to adjust your cooking accordingly. So if the red pepper is "too crunchy" the first time you try it, you might try roasting it for the next taste experiment.

7. **Rotate the new food into your family meals regularly.** How often will depend on your child; some will be open to new foods several times a week, whereas others may find that a little overwhelming at first.

Older children will be able to handle more variety (for example, raw red pepper in a salad one day, roasted red peppers another day), but younger children may prefer less variety. You know your child best!

8. **Keep trying! (the "Delicious Dozen" rule).** Don't give up if the food is rejected once, or twice, or even more often than that! Be persistent (but not insistent). The new food in question should reappear on your family menu regularly until your child learns to like it. If they don't like it, don't react. Instead, tell them "You're still learning to like it" or "You'll like that when you're a bit more grown-up" or "You just haven't tasted it enough times yet." It's important that older children, in particular, give new foods a chance. Remind them that children need to taste (some) new foods up to a dozen times before they become familiar enough to be eaten—our family calls this the "Delicious Dozen" rule. Kids love to count (particularly younger kids)! Even older ones like the challenge of remembering how many times they've tasted something.

Of course, you can adapt taste testing in any way that works for your family. One of my test family moms, Stacy, tried introducing new foods as a snack instead of a meal. Stacy found that this made taste testing more casual. With less pressure, she had better results with her 6- and 4-year-old boys. One day, for example, Stacy handed her kids a raw cranberry at snack-time, without any pressure to try it. They each took a bite! They tasted the cranberries again at afternoon snack the next day, after they had been dusted with sugar. That evening, Stacy added some dried cranberries to their dinner salad and they ate them all up!

Martha had a similar success. After months of trying—without success—to get 3-year-old Tobias to eat potatoes, she decided to try a taste-testing approach. She bought very small new pota-toes, which are a little sweeter than the large potatoes she usually bought. She served them whole, as usual. "They look cute," said Tobias. Previously, Martha had served the potatoes already peeled and mashed them for Tobias on his plate. But this time, Tobias and Martha peeled them together at the table, and Tobias mashed them himself on his plate. Result? "Oh, Mommy, I love them!"

A family food challenge: Four weeks, four new foods

After your child has learned the basics of taste testing, you can try introducing new foods regularly. The recipes that start on page 211 are designed to make this easy for children of all ages. For exam-ple, kids of any age will enjoy the Amazing Avocado Smoothie (page 300), which also works well for babies. As your baby grows, the recipes become more complex: you can serve the Avocado Smoothie to your baby, Beginner's Guacamole (page 301) to your toddler, and then Avocado Salsa Salad (page 304) to older children and adults. For older children who are cautious eaters, you can go back to the start, introducing these recipes in sequence: start with the smoothie; when they like that, follow up with the guacamole; and eventually, when they're ready, introduce the Avocado Salsa Salad—not forgetting the Awesome Avocado Ice Pops (page 303)! All of the recipes are designed to be used in a similar way: they can "grow" along with your child or be used in sequence to intro-duce older children to new foods and tastes.

How quickly should you try introducing each new food? I recommend creating a taste-testing plan, trying one new veget-able at a time. Most of my test families found that one vegetable per week was a good pace. Some families (with younger or more cautious kids) tried the same recipe multiple times. Other fam-ilies (with older or more adventurous kids) tried different recipes using the same vegetable. The recipes are organized by veg-etable, and there are four options per veggie—lots to choose from!

Vegetable	Taste Test 1	Taste Test 2	Taste Test 3	Taste Test 4
Broccoli	Recipe: Our thoughts:	Recipe: Our thoughts:	Recipe: Our thoughts:	Recipe: Our thoughts:
Carrots	Recipe: Our thoughts:	Recipe: Our thoughts:	Recipe: Our thoughts:	Recipe: Our thoughts:
Cauliflower	Recipe: Our thoughts:	Recipe: Our thoughts:	Recipe: Our thoughts:	Recipe: Our thoughts:
Green beans	Recipe: Our thoughts:	Recipe: Our thoughts:	Recipe: Our thoughts:	Recipe: Our thoughts:

Your family taste-testing plan

It might seem silly to have a formal taste-testing plan, but many children enjoy it. One of my taste-testing dads, Jon, printed the plan out and put it on a clipboard with a pen. His teenage children were impressed and took the exercise more seriously! Roberta posted her worksheet on the fridge, and her three boys (3, 5, and 7) loved writing down (with some help) their thoughts about the recipes. Opposite you will find an example of what to include. You can download a printable version of this worksheet at **GettingToYum.com**.

Four Fun games

These games introduce basic ideas about taste buds in order to give children a deeper understanding of their sense of taste. If your child is keen, you can try all four games. Otherwise, I recommend picking the most age-appropriate game that you think will interest your child the most.

Game 1:
The Five Senses (Ages 4 and up)

The main message: This game is designed to help your child get excited about learning about food through investigating the five senses: sight, touch, hearing, smell, and taste. This will allow your child to better understand their reactions to foods (both ones they like and ones they don't like). Ideally, play this at snack-time (when they are hungry, but not too hungry).

What you'll need: One of your child's preferred foods (ideally a fruit or vegetable).

What to do: Pick a food you know your child likes to eat—a favorite fruit or vegetable is ideal—and wash and prepare it together. For example, if you were to pick an apple, you might core and slice it.

Sit down with your child and let them know you're going to play a snack-time game. Let them see that you're excited and interested in their reaction. Then ask your child this series of questions. Be positive and encouraging no matter how they answer, and feel free to change the dialogue to fit your needs.

- Which foods do you like to eat?
- *Show them the food, then ask:* Which part of your body do you use to see?
- *Show them the food again, then ask:* What do you see?
- Which part of your body do you use to smell?
- *Ask them to smell the food, then ask:* What do you smell?
- Which part of your body do you use to touch?
- *Let them touch the food, then ask:* What does it feel like?
- *Encourage them to use words by asking follow-up questions about texture. For example:* Is it smooth or bumpy? Is it hot or cold? Is it sticky?
- *Ask them to "test" the food by tasting it, and then ask:* What does it taste like? *Encourage them to use words like sweet, salty, sour, crunchy, and so on.*
- What noise do you hear when eating it?
- *Once the child is done, ask:* How does your mouth feel now? Does it still taste like that food?

Repeat the game with other foods your child likes until they're comfortable with it. Then repeat this exercise with a new food your child has recently learned to like or with a new food that you believe they are quite likely to enjoy. Don't ask them to eat the food, but just to test it (which could mean simply licking it or putting it in their mouth to chew without necessarily swallowing). It's best if you make your initial taste-testing choices simple: a piece of dried or fresh fruit, for example. Gradually, repeat the game with more and more complex or "difficult" foods. Remember, don't judge their reactions! Simply ask them to describe the food. Be as curious as you hope they will learn to be.

Make sure to talk about it!

Many test families found that this game worked wonders with their younger children. The key is to ask kids to talk about the experience. As children do this, they learn to observe their reactions rather than simply to react to anything new in a negative, knee-jerk way. As you encourage your child's natural curiosity, they'll grow more confident about taste testing. Respect their opinions. If they don't like something, that's fine. Ask them to explain why (to the limits of their ability, of course). Over time, this game will help children become more open to trying new foods. Above all, make it fun!

Game 2:
The Five Flavors (Ages 4 and up)

The main message: This game introduces your child to the five different categories of flavors: sweet, salty, sour, bitter, and umami (savory)—which roughly translates from Japanese as "deliciously yummy." Umami is best described as a round, pleasant, savory or meaty or stock-like taste; it is found naturally in some fish and shellfish, certain vegetables (such as mushrooms, ripe tomatoes, spinach, and *kombu* seaweed), fermented, dried, and aged foods (including cured meats, green tea, Parmesan cheese, soy sauce, and balsamic vinegar), and also in the food additive MSG. Many classic food combinations maximize umami: Parmesan with tomato sauce, French fries with ketchup. (Breast milk apparently also has a relatively strong umami taste!)

What you'll need:

¼ teaspoon sugar or substitute of your choice (sweet)

¼ teaspoon sea salt (salty)

1 slice fresh lemon (sour)

1 small chunk unsweetened chocolate or 1 thin slice lemon peel (bitter)

1 thin slice Parmesan cheese (umami)

A glass of water

What to do:
Sample the different tastes. Place each of the five different food samples on a plate in front of your child. Place an identical plate in front of yourself. Make sure you each have a glass of water to rinse your mouth with in between each sample. Start with whichever sample your child is most interested in trying. One by one, taste each sample. (If your child is reluctant to taste anything, don't worry. Ask them to simply touch each sample with their tongue—putting a bit on a spoon helps!)

Discuss what you've tasted. Encourage your child to name the tastes. Your child will probably be surprised by the bitter taste of the unsweetened chocolate. Discuss why chocolate normally tastes sweet, and how sugar masks the bitter taste.

Chat about tastes at mealtimes. Remind your child of the different tastes when they encounter them at mealtimes; for example, discuss "sour" tastes if you serve grapefruit in a fruit salad. Encourage your child to incorporate "sweet," "salty," "sour," "bitter," and "umami" into their descriptions of tastes, foods, and meals. You'll find that your child's perceptions will start to change; for example, they may start to think of sour as an "interesting" rather than "yucky" taste.

Game 3:
Tasty Taste Buds (Ages 4 and up)

The main message: We're able to taste food because of our taste buds (the tiny bumps on our tongues and in our mouths). Taste buds are just like muscles: they can be trained! And some are weaker (or stronger) than others.

What you'll need:
A mirror
A magnifying glass

What to do:

Look at your tongue. Ask your child to look at their tongue in a mirror (a magnifying mirror, like those used for shaving, is great). Even better: have your child use a magnifying glass to look at your tongue or another family member's tongue. Ask your child to notice how the top of the tongue is bumpy and a bit rough-looking. Compare it to the underside, which is smoother. Explain that the bumps hold our taste buds. Older kids might be interested in the scientific word: *papillae* (*puh-PILL-ay*). The sandpaper-like texture of *papillae* also helps to grip food and move it around while we chew.

Young children can have up to 10,000 taste buds. Babies are born with more taste buds than adults and can taste what their mother has been eating—even before birth![25] As we age, our taste buds slowly atrophy, and the number of taste buds decreases. So, teenagers have fewer taste buds than young children, and adults have fewer than teenagers. This is why some foods may taste stronger to children than to adults.

Look more closely at your taste buds. Now that you both know what they look like, ask your child to look at their taste buds in a mirror. Have them drink a bit of milk, then look again. Can they see their taste buds more clearly? Ask your child to point out where their taste buds are the biggest and smallest, and whether some areas of their tongue have more taste buds than others. Some people have many more taste buds than others (these people are sometimes called "supertasters"—see Game 4: The Supertaster Game below). Ask siblings and parents to drink a little milk and then have your child examine their taste buds, and then their own. Does one person seem to have more taste buds than the others?

Try cooling your tongue (for ages 5 and up). Now that your child knows what taste buds look like, it's time to start learning more about how they work. Cold foods and drinks can make taste buds less sensitive. Cold can literally numb your taste buds: if you suck on an ice cube before you eat a food you don't like, you won't notice the taste as much. Try having your child taste a lemon—sour! Then ask them to put their tongue in a very cold glass of ice water or to suck on a plain ice popsicle for a few seconds. Have your child taste the lemon again. Does it taste less sour than before? Talk about why: just like cold fingers can't feel as well, taste buds are less sensitive when they are cold.

A variation on this theme is to use a popsicle. Have your child try a sip of their favorite juice and then taste a popsicle made from that same juice (if possible, make your own with a home popsicle set, using the same juice). The frozen popsicle won't taste as sweet as the juice itself at room temperature.

Game 4:
The Supertaster Game (Ages 6 and up)

The main message: People are naturally more or less sensitive to tastes (see page 24 for a description of the three categories of tasters). In this game, your child will compare their taste buds (or, more precisely, the tiny bumps or *papillae* that house the taste buds on the tongue) with other people. The more *papillae* a person has, the more taste buds they have, and the more sensitive to taste they generally are. Kids will discover if they are more or less sensitive tasters, and that it may take more or less time for them to learn to like new foods, depending on which category of taster they fall into. Supertaster kids will feel reassured that it's natural for them to take a bit longer to get used to new tastes.

What you'll need:
Food coloring (green or blue works best)
Cotton swabs
Reinforcement rings for hole-punched paper (one per
    participant)
Magnifying glass

What to do:

Guess your taste sensitivity: Tell your child you'll be doing a fun experiment. Explain that you'll be comparing the number of taste buds each of you have on your tongue using food coloring. Since the *papillae* don't absorb the food coloring, they remain red or pinkish (or even slightly whitish) in color, which makes it easier for kids to count the dots on their tongues. Explain to your child that you'll be using a simple measuring device (a reinforcement ring for hole-punched paper). On average, lower sensitivity tasters will have fewer than 15 *papillae* within the small circle, while supertasters may have twice that amount. Average tasters will be somewhere in the middle. Ask your child to guess whether they are an "average taster," a "supertaster," or a "low-sensitivity taster." (For younger children, you can just ask them to guess whether they'll have a "little," "average" or "middle," or "a lot.")

Count your taste buds. After you have recorded your child's guess, use a cotton swab to apply some food coloring onto your child's tongue. Place a reinforcement ring on the colored area and count the raised reddish/pink dots within the ring. Note: you are actually counting the *papillae*, on which the (much) smaller taste buds—which can't be seen by the naked eye—are clustered. Use a magnifying glass to help you! Double-count to check for accuracy. If you're really keen, you can compare the left and right sides of the tongue. Chances are that you'll have a lower number of *papillae* than the child—particularly on the tip of your tongue.[26] Interestingly, conventional wisdom used to be that distinct regions of the tongue were sensitive to different tastes (for example, the tongue is most sensitive to salt at the front, to sweet on the sides near the front, and to sour on the sides near the back). However, researchers have recently revisited—and are hotly debating—this issue. The only point on which they currently seem to agree is that all areas of the tongue are somewhat sensitive to all of the tastes.

Talk about it. Your child will have lots of questions about this experiment. Here are a few questions you might ask: Was your prediction correct? What would happen if you had fewer taste buds—would food taste less strong? What if you had more taste buds: would you be more sensitive? Is this why it takes longer for sensitive tasters to get used to eating new foods? Ask your child to list some positive aspects of each type of taster. For example, non-tasters will get used to new foods easily and are less likely to be bothered by new foods. Supertasters might be able to detect whether food is spoiled more easily.

Top Tips For Learning to Like New Foods

- **Taste (and love of healthy foods) can be taught.** This is a basic skill that all children can learn.
- **Don't label your child a picky eater; they're "learning to like" new foods.** Remind your child that practice makes perfect. This is empowering for children, and calming for parents. With practice and repeated exposure, children can learn to appreciate lots of different foods. Tell this to your child—and remind yourself regularly! Your job is to make these foods available; your child's job is to gradually familiarize themselves with these foods. Some kids will take longer than others, so be patient.
- **For most children, pickiness is not a personality trait; it is a *phase* that they'll get over.** Neophobia—the universal fear of new foods that emerges around the age of 2—is normal. Most children will go through a picky phase. *But this is only a phase.* Parents can help their child avoid this phase, or move through it more quickly, by helping them overcome their fear of new foods.
- **While all children *can* learn to eat a wide variety of foods, some will take longer than others** (just as some

take longer to learn to read than others). There *are* differences between children. Some are generalized (for example, girls tend to have more taste buds than boys), and some are specific (for example, some children will truly have more sensitive taste buds than others). Be patient! Practice makes perfect.

- **Introduce your child to new foods before you serve them.** When children say "I don't like that food," they often mean "I don't know it." Showing them the food prior to eating it helps increase familiarity, and thus acceptance.

- **Take "no" for an answer if your child has had one bite.** If you use force or pressure, it will backfire. Be as calm as possible and make sure to offer the food again another day.

- **It's important to start young, if you can.** Beyond making it an easier process, researchers now suggest that dieting and eating disorders—which have been viewed as problems that emerge during adolescence—are also influenced by events prior to puberty, linked to parents' own eating habits, weight issues, and parental child-feeding practices.[27]

- **It's not too late if your child is older.** The taste-training games are a fun way to help your child become more familiar with foods and help them understand their physical reactions. The recipes in the second half of the book are designed as a "ladder" to help your child move from simple to complex tastes and textures and to tame new foods along the way.

- *Believe* **that your child can learn to eat, and like, all kinds of food.** Expect your child to develop a more adventurous palate and—eventually—they will, particularly if you model this yourself! This can take time, so be patient.

Secret 2

Marketing Healthy Food to Your Kids Really Works!

Does yogurt grow on trees? Do sheep make eggs?

In a recent survey of 1000 British primary school students, fewer than 1 in 4 knew that beef burgers came from cattle. Some said that eggs came from sheep. Others said that cheese came from butterflies. Fewer than 2 in 3 knew that potato chips are made with potatoes.[1] Admittedly, these kids were relatively young. But even older children were found to have similar beliefs (my favorite: only 1 in 3 British teenagers correctly identified the sources of bacon, eggs, and milk).[2] Studies in Australia yielded comparable results: when asked where yogurt came from, 1 in 4 Australian children thought it grew on trees. When shown a drawing of a lunch box with bread, cheese, and a banana, less than half of Australian students could identify all three items as coming from farms.[3] One in 5 thought pasta came from an animal.

These examples are symptoms of food illiteracy: kids simply don't recognize an appropriate variety of foods, especially fruits and vegetables. More worryingly, even if children do have a high level of food and nutritional knowledge, they're not eating as well as they should.

The good news is that children can acquire food literacy pretty easily. Celebrity chef Jamie Oliver found this out while filming his hit TV show *Food Revolution* at a school in West Virginia. During the episode, a smiling Jamie places a bag on a desk in front of the kindergarteners, pulling vegetables out one by one. It's a cute scene, but something troubling quickly becomes apparent: the kids have no idea what *any* of the vegetables are. For cauliflower, one child bravely guesses "broccoli?" When shown a beet, the class is perplexed—another child ventures "celery?" Other children suggest that the eggplant Jamie proffers is a turnip, or a

pear. A series of increasingly more desperate *"What's this?"* questions from Jamie culminates in the scene's climax: he holds up a
bunch of ripe tomatoes. Surely, the kids will know what these are?
After a painful silence, one brave child raises his hand and asks,
"Are those potatoes?" Jamie then shows them two potatoes, and
the class falls silent. "We use potatoes to make french fries, did
you know that?" he asks. "No!" reply the children, most shaking
their heads. In the scene's (depressing) finale, Jamie pulls out
boxes of chicken nuggets, pizza, french fries, and hamburgers.
The kids all give immediate, enthusiastic replies—they know
exactly what these foods are (and it's clear that they like them).

The look on the teacher's face says it all. Her students have
failed a test that she didn't even know she should have been
preparing them for. The bad news is this is not unusual. But the
good news is that kids can learn—and quickly. A few days later,
Jamie went back to the classroom. This time, the kids shouted
out the answers cheerfully—and correctly.

Why is "getting to know" your vegetables important? Because
eating well, as chef Cyril Lignac (France's answer to Jamie Oliver)
says, requires that children "tame" new vegetables. In other words,
they need to familiarize themselves (sort of like getting to know
a new friend). The importance of familiarity—and the time it
takes to develop it—is a key food education tactic. As I've pointed
out before, often when kids say "I don't like it," they mean "I don't
know it." Your job (as a parent or educator) is to help them get
to know those new foods—to become food literate. Once children have gotten to know these foods, healthy eating will more
easily follow.

Food literacy has two aspects: 1) Food knowledge: children
are able to recognize a wide variety of foods and enjoy a wide
variety of tastes. 2) Food awareness: children know where food
comes from and how eating connects them to their families and
communities. Without food literacy, our chances of countering
the growing child obesity epidemic—which now affects not only
wealthy countries, but also the majority of countries around the
world—may be slim (no pun intended).

How food marketing undermines food literacy

Our ability to teach our children to love healthy food has been increasingly undermined by food marketing, which is now a multi-billion-dollar industry, using techniques that have become increasingly sophisticated.[4] American kids, for example, are exposed to over 40,000 food ads per year—most of which are for fast food, cereal, and candy.[5] And these ads work: marketing has a measurable effect on increasing consumption (if it didn't, why would those food companies spend all of that money?).[6]

The message isn't only on TV, which is just the tip of the iceberg. Celebrity endorsements, product placement, discount pricing, and increased container sizes are all used to encourage increased consumption. (Those candy bars at the checkout in your local grocery store? It's no accident that they are right at kids' eye level.)

Food advertising has also moved online in a big way, as it's both cheaper and a means of exposing kids to more advertising than on TV. The majority of top websites used by children contain food marketing.[7] Other websites encourage kids to continue the "brand experience" after leaving the site (through screensavers or desktop logos). Food companies also use "adver-gaming," blurring the boundaries between games and advertising. In the game "Jell-O Jiggle It," kids can get a cube of Jell-O to dance. "Sour Fling" asks them to fling virtual Sour Patch Kids candies past obstacles. Or players can "lick" virtual lollipops in "Dum Dums Flick-A-Pop" (originally designed as "Lick-A-Pop," before Apple complained that iPhones could be damaged by too much saliva); the app has been downloaded 1.5 million times. A step up in complexity is "Candy Sports," in which players can hit baseballs at a Skittles logo, play basketball in an arena plastered with Life Savers Gummies, and kick footballs into a Starburst sign.[8] The self-explanatory "Cookie Dough Bites Factory" has been downloaded more than 3 million times.

Full-blown websites have more complex games, such as Nestlé's "Nesquik Imagination Station" (hosted by a cute rabbit character, with a quiz game and spacesuit-making guide) or the imaginary McWorld on HappyMeals.com (complete with tree-house games for younger kids—pick your own Mc-Avatar!—and a sci-fi movie and book series for older kids).[9] Sound silly? HappyMeals.com had 350,000 visitors in *one single month* in 2011.[10]

Marketers also target adolescents on popular social media sites (like Facebook and Twitter), via smartphones and viral marketing (such as videos meant to be shared with friends), and even through sophisticated techniques like downloadable widgets (small applications downloaded to a child's computer or phone that allow companies to deliver targeted ads to users and their friends). Many of these approaches target older children's and adolescents' developmental needs—such as bonding with peers and establishing their own identity—and are thus hard to resist, which makes them potentially more dangerous than traditional forms of advertising because they seek to elicit emotional responses and hence deep loyalty to brands.[11]

Of course, marketing is a legitimate business activity. If it encourages children to overeat unhealthy foods, however, it has both health and economic implications—particularly (although not only) obesity-related.[12] This issue is now of such concern to policy-makers in the US that Congress recently asked the top medical research agency in the country—the Center for Disease Control and Prevention—to study the link between obesity and food marketing to children. The resulting Institute of Medicine study, *Food Marketing to Children and Youth: Threat or Opportunity*, makes for chilling reading.[13] The report found that food marketing intentionally targets children who are too young to distinguish between truth and advertising. Researchers now believe that the effects of marketing on our subconscious, automatic behaviors are widespread and long lasting.[14] By watching these ads, our children may literally be programmed for a lifetime of unhealthy eating.[15]

The report also documents the tactics used by food marketing companies to make their messages compelling. Food marketing companies conduct extensive research on children—even preschoolers. To improve their ability to leverage children's suggestibility, they explore the psychological underpinnings of children's food choices, probing and testing "child archetypes" (to get their spokes-characters just right), and figuring out ways to help kids leverage or subvert the "psyche of mothers as the family gatekeeper." Marketing strategies have proliferated, and gotten subtler, targeting "cool" messages at some age groups and "cute" messages at others, until heavily marketed brands become central to children's sense of identity and self.[16] Scary.

Of course, marketers argue that advertising is free speech and that marketing is good for business. Those same arguments were used for cigarette marketing in the past—and are arguments we should no longer accept, as Marion Nestle has brilliantly argued in her book *Food Politics*.[17] But the power of the food industry is such that the regulatory controls that exist in some countries—like France, where vending machines, fast food, and food advertising of any kind are banned in all schools—are far from universal.

So what's a parent to do? Of course, you can reduce your kids exposure to marketing messages. Even simply setting limits on screen time has been shown to be beneficial for kid's health.[18] This is, in part, because exposure to TV food advertising (with its "snacking = enjoyment" messages) increases calories consumed during and immediately afterward—whether or not kids are actually hungry.[19] (This is true for adults, too, by the way.)

I realize that turning off the TV isn't likely to make you a popular parent. Luckily, there are positive things you can do. One of the most powerful strategies of all turns marketing on its head: *you* can market food to your kids.

You can market food to your kids!

Cornell University marketing guru Brian Wansink has spent decades finding ways to market healthy food to kids. His idea is simple: why not invert the logic of food marketers, which masterfully induce cravings for processed foods and junk foods of all kinds? This sounded like a tall task: how could academic researchers, no matter how savvy, take on marketing companies with huge advertising budgets?

Wansink's strategy was ingenious in its simplicity. He found that renaming vegetables with silly (or branded) names worked wonders with kids. His team served "X-ray Vision Carrots" and "Power Punch Broccoli" along with "Tiny Tasty Tree Tops" and "Silly Dilly Green Beans." They tested this out in a few schools (including two in New York) with amazing results: up to 100 percent increased consumption of vegetables![20] Another experiment by Wansink's team found that preschoolers were more likely to make healthy choices if foods were visually branded with sympathetic figures.[21]

Wansink also developed an experiment for older kids, specifically focused on healthy choices in fast food restaurants. This is admittedly a tough nut to crack: even though many fast food restaurants now offer healthy choices, few kids pick them. Realistically, how many kids are going to choose a side salad instead of fries (even if offered Newman's Own Balsamic Vinaigrette?). And would apple dippers really beat a vanilla ice-cream cone? Not for most kids.

Wansink was convinced that something *could* be done to help kids make healthy choices. His research team designed an experiment that would prime kids through the power of suggestion and association.[22] The experiment was simple: kids at a summer camp, ranging from 6 to 12 years old, were asked to participate in the study. They were invited to go out for a fast food lunch once per week, four weeks in a row. (I'm thinking it wasn't very hard to convince kids to sign up for this experiment!)

At each lunch, each child was given a choice between french fries and apple dippers. The first week, kids were simply asked what they wanted, without any attempt to influence their choices. The second week, however, kids were asked to complete a brief questionnaire, privately, before going to the restaurant. Researchers showed each child pictures of six superheroes and asked them what the superhero would eat: apples or fries? Kids were then asked what their own choice would be. The next week, kids were shown several pictures of healthy foods (including fries and apples), and then were asked to classify the foods as healthy or unhealthy. Again, after the exercise, the kids were asked to choose between french fries and apple dippers. The result? In the first week, only 1 in 10 kids picked the apple slices. After being asked about superhero choices, nearly 5 out of 10 children (*half* the kids) picked apples.

I appreciated Wansink's insights when we were over at my cousin's house for dinner one night. A fairly zealous whole foods sort of person (without kids), she had prepared a wonderful dinner that featured braised kale and pearl barley. As she proudly served them, my daughters stared at their plates for a few seconds while I watched, wondering what to do (they'd never had pearl barley before). Meanwhile, the smell of the barley—a yeasty fresh-bread-just-out-of-the-oven sort of smell—wafted over the table.

"It smells like bread!" exclaimed Claire. I had my eureka moment.

"What's that?" Sophie cautiously asked, fidgeting and ever so slowly sliding her plate away from her.

"Oh, that's Fairy Baguette!" I said cheerfully, sliding the plate back toward her. "Fairies are tiny and this is just their size!"

Sophie looked dubious, but Claire took the bait.

"Fairy Baguette! Yum!" she chirped, before picking up a grain of barley and nibbling on it. "It's delicious! Try some!" And her older sister did just that.

Of course, you don't have to use only child-friendly names to work your marketing magic. The French tend to use place-based names for dishes.[23] Often, those names relate to the places where the food is from, with a regional *terroir* ("taste of place") emphasis that is so characteristic of French family cuisine. *Carottes Vichy* (see page 225) is a divine, melt-in-your-mouth carrot dish (and super easy to make) that conjures up images of traditional cuisine from one of France's heartlands. Or think of the classic beef bourguignon, which comes from Burgundy, southeast of Paris, one of the most famous gastronomic regions of France. Or what about the dessert favorite *Poires Belle Hélène* (see page 336), invented by renowned chef Escoffier, named after a 19th-century opera by Offenbach (this is the equivalent of naming a dish after a blockbuster movie!). Avatar Asparagus? Harry Potter Hash Browns? Lion King Lettuce! You get the idea.

The take-home message is simple: appealing names work wonders. Families often find that this is a nice alternative to the sneaky chef method: renaming foods (rather than hiding them) allows kids to get over their food fears. One of our French friends, Virginie, loves to tell the story about "sea chicken" (*poule de mer*): her older daughter Emma didn't like fish, but loved chicken. So Virginie hit on the idea of serving relatively mild, white fish (like sole) and calling it "sea chicken." It took years before Emma liked fish, but she never once balked at her *poule de mer* dish.

Another simple experiment one of my test families tried was with potatoes. Kristine's 2- and 5-year-old girls refused to eat potatoes, flat out. They'd been that way since they started solids. I suggested something that I'd tried when my younger daughter, Claire, balked at eating potatoes: renaming them "volcanoes"! The approach is simple: mash up a boiled potato into a cone shape, poke a small hole in the top, stick a little piece of butter in the top, and watch the butter melt and run down the sides like (you guessed it) lava. Here's what Kristine had to say:

> On your advice, at Thanksgiving dinner I mounded the potatoes, made a hole in the top, and poured in the gravy, then told the girls in an excited tone that they were eating "potato volcanoes"! The girls ate every bite! This idea is pure genius.
>
> —Kristine

The power of parent-led marketing

One of the most powerful ways to market food to children is to use parental role modeling. If parents (or other trusted caregivers) are seen to eat a food and enjoy it, kids are much more likely to try it and to report that they liked it. This parental effect was even more pronounced with younger children.[24] The families that offered new foods in a loving, calm environment achieved the best results. In one experiment, children were given the option of eating a sandwich with a new and unfamiliar filling alone or while sitting with their mother and having a quiet but social time together. Children who chose the latter option (and the majority did) not only liked the new filling more at the end of the six-week experiment, they were also more likely to try other new foods.[25]

My test families report that teaching children to like new foods often means that parents have to change their cooking and eating habits. Remember 3-year-old Lucas? When his parents began taste training, his mother, Jessica, realized that it might help if she started to do some of the cooking (her husband had been doing most of it). "I realized that the reason the only meat Lucas liked to eat was hot dogs was that it was the only kind of meat I felt comfortable cooking," she confessed. With encouragement from her husband, Jessica tried out a variety of easy vegetable recipes (all included in the second part this book) and found—to her delight—that there are vegetables Lucas actually loves, including ones that Jessica herself had trouble eating as a child. Most important, reports Jessica, "I think it's great that Lucas sees his mom in the kitchen—it helps to illustrate how important food is to us, and how much we enjoy it!"

The Me Too Method

One of the fun twists on parent-led marketing is something I call the "Me Too Method." The idea is simple: if you serve it to yourself and eat it with obvious enjoyment, children's natural curiosity will be piqued, and they'll be more likely to want some, too. I've tried this numerous times in the past, but recently decided to test this method again one night. After our main course, I served myself some lovely baby spinach salad, topped with vinaigrette and tiny little pieces of mandarin orange. I didn't say a word to the kids, but calmly kept chatting to my husband about our day. My younger daughter Claire—who is not the world's most enthusiastic salad eater—looked up at me and said, "Why didn't *I* get any salad?" Sophie, never one to like being left out, followed suit. They both promptly proceeded to eat a plateful of salad.

Christine, one of my readers, used this approach to great effect with her toddler, who was having a hard time learning to like yogurt. In fact, Christine barely had time to put yogurt down on the table before the "no yogurt!" refrain would be heard. One day she decided to try something different. Instead of a plastic tub, Christine put a new, small glass bowl on the table. "Look! Look at your beautiful new tasting bowl!" Her toddler examined it with great intrigue and watched as Christine placed a dollop of pink (raspberry) yogurt into it, saying, "Here's a tiny taste for you." Christine then proceeded to eat a spoonful of her own, savoring it with lots of "mmmm" and "yum," obviously relishing the sweet taste. After a moment, her toddler grabbed her own spoon and popped a bit of yogurt into her mouth. Then, with obvious delight, the little hand darted out again and again, until she cleaned her bowl. "I took a taste!" was her proud response. Now yogurt is a favorite in Christine's house.

The "why" of eating: It's *not* about nutrition

Marketing food to your kids isn't just a playful distraction. It's actually a crucial contribution to their eating success. Research shows that food *preferences* (not nutritional knowledge) play an important role in enabling children (and adults) to make healthy food choices.[26] In other words, we eat what we *like* to eat, even if we know it's not good for us. We avoid eating what we don't like to eat, even if we know it *is* good for us.

In fact, nutritional information can backfire. Dr. Marion Nestle

argues that many of us suffer from nutrition confusion: conflict-
ing, competing, and rapidly changing nutrition claims that confuse
consumers, increase anxiety, and encourage us to buy over-
processed foods on the basis of (at times) dubious nutritional
claims. Because of this, many nutritionists now recommend a
different, simpler idea: the greater variety of foods (including
fruits and vegetables) a child eats, the wider range of nutrients
they will get.

Your goal is to get your child eating a variety of foods.
Marketing healthy foods to your child helps them establish the
right food preferences. If you just worry about nutrition,
you're fighting a losing battle. Instead of telling your child
"Eat this, it's good for you," try telling them "Eat this, it tastes
good!"

> *At dinner tonight, instead of saying "You have to eat
> this," I kept saying "Yum, it's delicious!" My 3-year-old
> kept laughing and repeating it—and ate her entire dinner
> without a complaint. I'm not exaggerating—she's really
> changed her approach overnight."*
>
> —*Françoise*

In other words, *telling* your child to eat a variety of foods so
that they get nutrients isn't a great strategy for success. Enabling
them to eat these foods because they truly believe they are
yummy will, for most kids, work better. And vitamins and
minerals are better absorbed from fresh food rather than from
vitamin pills.[27] When I asked our family doctor in France whether
Claire was getting enough iron and needed iron supplements,
he looked at me curiously and then laughed. "Get her to eat
parsley and beets!" was his calm response.

I'll admit that getting children to eat a variety of nutrient-rich
foods often requires parents to be inventive—but it can also be fun!
I remember the time our friends Sonja and Jamie visited us with
their daughter, Carrie, a feisty 2-year-old and rigidly picky eater
who at that time was eating only scrambled eggs and buttered

toast—for breakfast, lunch, and dinner. Despite their efforts, green vegetables in any form would not pass this child's lips.

"She won't eat anything but scrambled eggs," her mother told us, evidently consigned to her child's fate (with Carrie in the room, who was quietly, but intently, listening). "You want to bet?" replied my husband, Philippe, who took this on as a personal challenge. After a bit of brainstorming, he took some of the rice we had cooked for dinner and mixed it in the food processor with some steamed spinach and a big dollop of honey. He poured the velvety smooth, melt-in-your-mouth, electric green purée into a little bowl with a cheerful cartoon on the bottom. Tiny dabs of butter decorated the top: two eyes, a nose, and a little button mouth.

"Look what we're eating! Spinach Surprise!" announced Philippe, with just a little bit of a flourish. As he handed the bowl to Carrie he said in a firm, inviting voice, "There's a *surprise* at the bottom of *your* bowl—but only yours!" The rest of us were handed normal white bowls, and we dipped our spoons in without comment (her parents having been instructed to say nothing and to continue our dinner conversation as if nothing out of the ordinary was happening).

At first, Carrie looked mutinous. She stared at her bowl. Her bowl stared back at her. (As instructed, we all stared at our bowls, too, and then started eating.)

"Quick—the eye is melting!" joked my husband. He popped Carrie's spoon into the bowl, nestling it just under the dab of butter in question—which now looked quite teary-eyed, as the butter melted in a little transparent yellow streak. He turned away to continue his conversation.

Out of the corner of my eye, I saw Carrie take a quick look around the table, scowling. Not getting any attention, her eyes strayed to her bowl. After a minute's hesitation, she tentatively lifted the spoon to her mouth and oh-so-delicately licked the tee-niest, tiniest bit of buttery spinach. Thoughtfully, she licked her lips, casting her eyes around the table. Nobody, it seemed, was paying attention. Then the spoon reached down for the other "eye." And then the nose, then the mouth ... until Carrie had scraped the bowl clean and found the cartoon hiding at the bottom of her bowl.

Carrie is now a healthy, athletic teenager who eats pretty much everything (including spinach). How did she get there? First, lots of practice! Her parents exposed her to vegetables over and over again, in lots of different ways. Second, creativity: they figured out which recipes, cooking strategies, and presentation (including fun names) worked best for their family. Third, they made family meals fun.

Note that I didn't mention nutritional information. Do you really think that a toddler who can't yet count to 100 is going to be motivated to eat their spinach because it's "high in iron"? You know that your kids should eat certain foods, but using nutritional information to encourage them is probably not going to work. (In fact, it doesn't really work for most adults either!)

Tactics to avoid: When marketing backfires

Marketing food to kids works best when you adopt a positive approach. When you market healthy foods to your children, emphasize pleasure rather than the deprivation associated with diets or banning certain foods.

You can also teach your kids to seek out good foods that they enjoy (which I call "eat most of the time foods") rather than avoiding "bad" foods (which you can label "once in a while foods"). Try to avoid making your child feel guilty for enjoying treats. Avoiding negative emotional associations with food helps children avoid feelings of guilt that might translate into emotional eating and poor eating habits, and even eating disorders. After all, treats are fun—in moderation.

Although being positive is important, don't overdo the praise. A degree of praise can increase how much children perceive they enjoy (and actually consume) healthy foods, but too much praise can make children uncomfortable or even backfire.[28] Simple yet positive observations ("You enjoyed your meal, didn't you?" or "You did your best at tasting that new food") will make a child more comfortable than lavish praise (which might imply blame or parental anxiety if the child doesn't measure up).

Perhaps most important, don't use bribes or rewards. Research shows that these increase kids' preferences for the "reward" food (such as dessert) and decrease their preferences for the "required" food (such as salad).[29] Bribes and rewards might work in the short term, but they don't teach kids the right behaviors in the long term.

Marketing Food to your kids: Getting started

How can you put these marketing ideas into action? In addition to the ideas discussed in this chapter, here are four fun games that will teach your kids important concepts—such as how our sense of smell is related to taste—and will give you some sure-fire strategies for taking the fear out of new foods.

Game 5:
The Silly Name Game (Ages 3 and Up)

The main message: This fun game involves labeling foods with names that will ignite your child's enthusiasm for new foods. Using "superhero" or "silly" names might work for younger kids; stylish or "cool" names might work for older kids.

In case you're dubious, let me reassure you: everyone who has tried this game has told me that it works. Parents have so few fun, easy tactics in their arsenal that you shouldn't pass this one up! Moreover, there's a difference between being playful and playing with food. In the former case, you can be respectful of the food but still light-hearted about it. This game doesn't mean you allow kids to actually play with their food. Rather, you focus on putting them in a relaxed (rather than oppositional) mood, which makes mealtime easier. Remember that renaming strange foods in ways that make them familiar can help your kids get over the fear of new foods, making it easier for them to adapt (particularly when you're traveling or eating at other people's houses).

What you'll need: Imagination and a sense of humor!

What to do: Ask your child to name dishes (or name dishes in their honor if they help design or make them!). If you travel, try to sample at least one local dish; when you're back home, try making it and give it a name that refers to the place where you first ate it. Or try silly names—even with older kids. You might be surprised by how much they enjoy it!

When I asked other parents about the Silly Name Game, I got some great suggestions. Turns out that lots of parents already do this! Nina wrote to me to tell me that spinach is called Monster Surprise in her house. When introducing broccoli to her toddler, Brandy explained that broccoli buds were baby flower buds—and her toddler promptly renamed it "Broccoli Flowers," which she ate with gusto!

You can also use the power of association. You can apply this logic when eating out, using your child's favorite superhero (or just plain hero!). "What would Batman pick?" was used in the experiment described earlier in this chapter. "What would Dora pick?" would work in my younger daughter's case. Or, for older kids, pick a sports figure or celebrity—or someone you know personally that they look up to—who's known for healthy eating.

Game 6:
The Smell-Taste Experiment (Ages 6 and up)

The main message: This game teaches kids that our senses of smell and taste are related. It also helps them understand that smell plays a large part in determining how things taste. Kids will even learn how artificial flavors are used to fool our taste buds (the most fun part of this game!).

What you'll need:
3 lollipops of different flavors (but similar textures)
A blindfold

What to do:
Discuss the relationship between smell and taste. Ask your child to think about how smell and taste may be related. For example, ask your child if they have ever noticed how having a cold diminishes their sense of taste. Explain this is because their sense of smell is temporarily affected. For older children, you can explain the relationship between smell and taste in a bit more detail. Aromas are detected when odors (airborne molecules) pass through the nose and are absorbed by cells inside the nose. When the nose is blocked, the tongue will taste the sugar and acid, but not detect the lemon smell, for example. Smell thus enhances the taste of food by allowing us to combine complex aromas with the five basic tastes (described on page 41). Older kids may also enjoy learning new vocabulary. The word "olfaction" refers to our sense of smell. The word "gustation" refers to our sense of taste.

Plug your nose! Blindfold your child, ask them to plug their nose, and have them try each flavored lollipop, one after the other. Ask them to guess the flavor of each lollipop. This is way more difficult than you might expect!

Chat about flavors. Ask your child why they think food companies would use artificial flavors in food. You can explain that many artificial foods (such as candies) are made from similar ingredients and so have very similar tastes, and that it is the use of different scents or perfumes that makes them taste different. Many food companies employ flavorists (yes, this is a real job) to create these smell/taste combinations using edible chemicals and extracts that alter the flavor of food through influencing our sense of smell.

Game 7:
The Mystery Smell Game (Ages 6 and up)

The main message: This game introduces the idea that smells have strong emotional associations and often help us recall memories of places, people, or events. Children will experience how smell evokes memories and emotions and connect this to their feelings about food.

What you'll need:
A blindfold
Cotton balls
Containers, preferably plastic ones with lids
Four or five items with scents, including:

- Familiar smells (for example, perfume, shampoo, vanilla extract, lemon, banana, cinnamon)
- Pungent smells (for example, pine needles, vinegar, coffee, ginger, garlic, peppermint, curry powder)
- Hard-to-identify smells (for example, pencil shavings, dirt, olive oil, a slice of raw potato)

What to do:
Prepare the containers. Place a different item in each container (for liquids, soak a cotton ball and place that in the container). Tip: keep the items separated and the containers closed to prevent the odors from mixing.

Smell the items. Ask your child to put on the blindfold and then smell the containers one by one. Then ask your child to rate the odor: older kids can use more complex language (strong, neutral, pleasant, pungent); younger kids can simply say "good" or "bad."

Chat about it. Ask your child if they think a substance is edible or not (regardless of whether they correctly identify it). Ask your child to talk about any memories associated with the smells. You might be surprised by the responses! You can give your own examples (one brand of shampoo reminds me of summer camp, and a specific type of perfume always reminds me of my mom).

Game 8:
The Store Brand versus Name Brand Blind Taste Test (Ages 9 and Up)

The main message: Brands influence our perception of taste and quality. Even if the food doesn't taste better, our belief that it will (which is created by the branding) influences our sense of taste. This game helps children to think critically about their emotional responses to branding.

What you'll need: Pick at least two matching pairs of name-brand and store-brand items. Here's a list of potential pairs, taken from a *Consumer Reports* test of name-brand/store-brand pairs:[30]

Kellogg's Rice Krispies versus store-brand rice cereal
Skippy peanut butter versus store-brand peanut butter
Nature's Valley granola bars versus store-brand granola bars
Coca-Cola or Pepsi versus store-brand cola

What to do:
Chat about branding. Ask your child whether they think that brands influence their sense of taste. With older children, you can discuss how branding influences taste. For example, in one study kids liked the taste of foods more when they were presented in McDonald's packaging, compared with the identical foods without any branding.[31] In another experiment, children were shown an enjoyable ad for a new food and then tried the

food; they rated the new food tastier than those who tried the food before viewing the ad.[32] Studies with teens and adults have shown similar effects, like the famous blind taste test for name-brand cola versus store-brand cola.

Sample the blinded pairs. Ask your child to sample each pair of products and record their observations (what they liked and didn't like) and overall preferences. At the end, reveal their preferences and count up the number of choices of name-brand versus store-brand options.

Variation—The Switcheroo: Switch the labels on the name-brand and store-brand products. For example, you would put out the following, clearly labeled:

- One bowl of Rice Krispies cereal (labeled "store brand") and one bowl of store-brand rice cereal (labeled "Rice Krispies")
- One glass of name-brand cola (labeled "store brand") and one glass of store-brand cola (labeled with the name brand)

Ask your child to taste both samples and indicate which one they prefer, then reveal the switch!

Chat about the results. Has your child ever pestered you for a name-brand product and resisted the store brand? Ask them to think about why.

If you did the "switcheroo" experiment and your child preferred the store brand in the name-brand packaging, ask them why they thought this was the case. How much did their belief about the brand influence their expectations and actual taste experience?

An important point to discuss with your child is how much more the name-brand products cost versus the store-brand products. Is the extra money worth it? Why (or why not)?

Top Tips For Marketing Healthy Food to Your Kids

- **Talk less about health and more about good tastes.** Don't cajole with nutritional information (such as explanations that a food has a lot of iron or calcium). Instead, emphasize how delicious the food is. For example, try saying "Taste this, it's really yummy" rather than "Eat this, it's good for you." Tell your children that good-for-you foods taste good. Healthy eating habits will be a happy by-product. *"Broccoli? Yum!"*
- **Eat with your children, tasting foods with obvious enjoyment.** Are you modeling picky eating behavior for your children? If so, consider changing your own eating habits. Get other influential role models involved (like older peers) when possible.
- **Give dishes attractive (or silly) names.** Sound silly? The Silly Name Game (page 64) shows the contrary—it works, even on adults!
- **Don't use bribes or rewards.** Research shows that these increase kids' preferences for the "reward" food (such as dessert) and decrease their preferences for the "required" food (such as salad).[33]
- **Do use moderate praise.** A recent study showed that social praise actually increased intrinsic liking for and consumption of healthy foods among children over a 3-month period.[34] (But don't overdo it—it may backfire.)
- **Don't label foods as "good" or "bad."** Call foods "eat most of the time" foods and "occasional treats." Teach your child the difference, and don't make them feel guilty for enjoying treats—that way you'll avoid emotional eating.
- **Teach your kids to seek out good foods they enjoy (rather than avoiding "bad" foods).** The difference is subtle but important. Healthy eating is about pleasure, not deprivation.

Secret 3

Schedule One Snack a Day

Ask any parent whether they pack food when leaving home with their kids, and chances are that they're hoarding snacks. Crisps, snack bars, juice and more are tucked away in pockets, glove compartments, and bags for that inevitable moment when children declare they are hungry. The cozy, even comforting, image of snack-time is a cliché of childhood. Kids need to snack, right? Tiny tummies need filling up at regular intervals, right? Even if they didn't, the prospect of a food deprivation-induced tantrum is more than many parents can bear. Anyway, why would you deprive a child of their snack? With kids, it's normal that snack-time is pretty much all the time, isn't it?

Well, it turns out that this behavior is normal in North America—and to a lesser extent in the UK—but not (at least traditionally) in many other places. In China, snacking is rare, and foods consumed as snacks (such as rice crackers) are low in calories.[1] In Italy, meals are eaten three times a day, with only one snack—a mid-afternoon snack called the *merenda*. The same is true in France, where children as young as 2 years old happily subsist on four meals a day: breakfast, lunch, dinner, and a scheduled afternoon snack (actually more like a mini-meal) known as the *goûter* (goo-*tay*). Of course, cultural norms for eating differ greatly from one country to the next, but it seems safe to say that prior to the advent of industrial food culture, snacking used to be relatively rare—both because of constraints (lack of income; the time and expense needed to gather and prepare foods; lack of ability to ship and store prepared foods) and folk wisdom about regulating one's eating habits.

The modern "snack-time all the time" phenomenon is, it turns out, relatively recent. Snacking rates rose rapidly from the 1970s onward, along with the rise of processed food and the food marketing industry.[2] Back in the 70s, North American children snacked once a day (and a quarter of kids didn't snack at all). Today, North American kids snack on average three times a day; and one in five children snacks five times a day or more.[3] (A significant proportion of adults also snack multiple times per day.[4]) And they're not alone: children in many countries—from England to Australia to India to Mexico—have jumped on the snacking bandwagon.[5]

The increase in snacking is one of the major causes of increasing child obesity rates.[6] As much as we wish otherwise, most kids aren't snacking on apples and carrots. Salty snacks, fizzy drinks, and candy are the most popular choices—and biggest calorie jolts. Snacks are the source for more than 1 in 4 calories that our kids now consume. At the same time, fewer children are eating three regular meals per day. Snacks are substituting for breakfast or even lunch—with some schools even going so far as to replace lunchtime with "snack breaks" or "nutrition breaks" to save time during the school day.

However, most doctors and other medical experts argue that frequent snacking is a bad idea because kids often aren't hungry enough to eat the nutritious foods served at mealtimes. That's not all: since adult food habits are formed during childhood, excessive snacking teaches our kids poor eating habits. Feeding kids typical snack foods fosters taste preferences for poor-quality foods of little nutritional value. Most processed snack food is engineered to achieve precisely this result, with addictive combinations of fat, sugar, and salt that are designed to keep us coming back for more.[7] Snacking leads us to overeat while (ironically) decreasing our overall intake of nutrients. Simply put: kids don't need to snack. They might *want* to, but they don't *need* to.

The assertion that kids don't need more than one snack per day is controversial. On the one hand, some parents argue that regular snacking has benefits (balancing out blood glucose levels, for example). Some snacking supporters argue that "grazing" (random snacking) is fine, as long the foods being consumed are healthy. Other parents disagree. They argue that random snacking might be fine when your preschooler has a choice between cucumbers and carrots at home, but not so desirable when kids hit high school, with access to vending machines and fast food. Others argue that unrestricted snacking creates a deregulated approach to eating that might work for a toddler, but not as a life-long approach to eating.

One fact seems clear: if eating any time or all the time becomes normal, children risk developing a habit of eating even when they aren't hungry.[8] And if snacking is used to regulate children's behavior (in response to crankiness, for example), this creates the risk of allowing your child to develop emotional eating behaviors. Bored? Why not go to the cupboard and rummage around for something? Tired? Here, have some crackers!

The best way to avoid emotional eating is by scheduling meals and snacks; this takes emotions and impulsive eating out of the equation. That's not all: studies show that scheduling snacking reduces obesity rates.[9] But what schedule will work best? Most experts recommend allowing children to snack at most twice a day (and preferably, for kids 6 and up, only once per day).[10] Make sure to schedule three predictable, nutritious, filling meals per day. For children under 5, offer two snacks a day: one in mid-morning and one in mid-afternoon. For children 5 and older, offer one snack a day, usually in the mid- to late afternoon. This routine may evolve as your children grow, participate in sports, and so on. For teenagers, try increasing the size of their meals and snack rather than adding more snacks to their routine.

Many of my test families had great results by creating a snacking routine. Heidi wrote to me to explain how well this snacking routine was working for their family after I posted some ideas on my blog:

> *The snack thing has been way out of control in our house. I had never thought about the snacking as having any negative effects. We only offer healthy snacks, and the North American view that children need to eat*

frequently and that many small meals are healthier than three big ones had led me not to question the snacking habit. After deciding to follow the "one snack per day" approach, I tracked what the kids ate for a few days and realized they were eating much less protein and vegetables than I realized because of all the fruit, crackers, muffins, smoothies, and granola bars they were eating as snacks all day! Often the kids weren't hungry for dinner, ate only half of it, and then got more snacks later. The eating on the go, the crumbs, the mess, the snack containers going missing! We've now eliminated snacks to one substantial after-school snack, and it has made a huge difference in how much dinner the kids eat! They are also not hungry for bedtime snacks, either. I love this!

—Heidi

Pediatrician Nimali Fernando, who blogs under the name "Doctor Yum," also wrote to me with her thoughts. Nimali confessed she wasn't different from many moms. She carried snacks "just in case" (what if someone has a meltdown? what if the family is stuck somewhere without food?), and their kitchen counter featured a big snack basket, which her kids invariably dipped into right before dinner. Inspired by the "one snack per day" idea, Nimali tried her own experiment at home:

For the past month, I have instituted a "no snacking" and "le goûter" (afternoon snack) at my house, and I'm pleased to say it has worked brilliantly. During soccer season, our heartier goûter snack held the kids over until after practice, and the kids were much more able to eat a nutritious dinner that I served because they weren't munching in the car on the way home. The kids now understand the rules about snacking, and as long as they have plenty to do, they don't seem to miss snacks.

Nimali and her family learned an important lesson: mild hunger is a normal human sensation. If children's (and adults') stomachs are comfortably empty before mealtimes, they will be more likely to eat well. As Nimali summed it up, "A child who is faced with broccoli at dinner is more likely to eat it if she's not full of crackers and fruit snacks."

Just like Doctor Yum, when my daughters tell me they feel hungry, I don't necessarily feed them. I check in with our routine. If it's not time to eat, I tell them, "That's great, you'll really appreciate your next meal. It's in X hours." Sometimes the next meal is only an hour away, but sometimes it is two or three hours away. That's okay—they know they have to wait. My kids and I both know that we have a set routine in our house: three nutritious, energy-dense meals a day (at which they can eat as much or as little as they want), and one ample afternoon snack. This means that they eat as much as they feel they need at meals, and know they will be able to eat well at their next meal.

The difference between *Feeling* hungry and being hungry

Doctor Yum's story raises an important point: *It's okay for your child to feel a little bit hungry.* If they eat three meals and one nutritious snack per day, your child will not starve. Research shows that children intuitively compensate by eating more at mealtimes (provided, of course, that those mealtimes are scheduled and predictable).[11] By limiting snacks, you're enabling them to establish this internal regulation skill, whereby they can sense whether they're hungry or not. And by permitting them to snack all the time (or by offering overly large portions or calorie-laden sweet or salty snack foods) you are undermining this skill.[12]

No one wants a child to *be* hungry, but we seem to have extended the term "hungry" to include everything from feeling peckish to being malnourished. This is often associated with the habit of feeding kids as soon as (or even before) they let you know they're hungry. By doing so, parents miss an opportunity to teach their child a valuable skill: knowing what a comfortably empty stomach feels like. This skill allows children not to overeat and to wait comfortably until the next mealtime—a classic example of self-regulation.

How do you teach your child this approach? Simple: just don't let them randomly snack. If you do snack, schedule it. When you set up this schedule, explain to your child that "We only eat at mealtimes, and otherwise we can happily wait." Being happy with that feeling of a comfortably empty stomach will enable your child to wait patiently until their next meal—setting up good eating habits for life.

The French have an expression for this feeling of pre-meal hunger: they call it a *bonne maladie* (a "good illness"). This feeling, they tell their children, is a *good* feeling—kind of like that wonderful anticipation you feel in the run-up to your birthday. You wouldn't have your birthday party a week early, would you? There's nothing wrong with feeling a bit hungry if a nutritious and filling meal is going to be on the table soon.

Remember: don't feel panicked at the thought of your child feeling hungry (as opposed to truly *being* hungry). I know many parents might (I certainly did when we transitioned our daughters). One mom, Shaylagh, wrote to me about these fears. She confessed that she had become a "fear feeder," despite her best intentions. As Shaylagh noted, "I'd fill his belly to avoid conflict and then wonder why he was fussy at dinner." But after she established a meal and snack schedule, her toddler's behavior improved. No more negotiating, impulsiveness, or tantrums! Shaylagh had discovered one of the most helpful principles of parenting: children will behave well when the rules are known and followed consistently because they're confident their needs will be met in a timely and satisfying fashion.

The art of anticipation: Teaching patience

Scheduling snacks is a great way to teach children patience. Or, rather, to frame patience as "the art of anticipation" (doesn't that sound so much more appealing and positive?). While everyone is waiting for dinner, you can talk about the meal you're going to have, show your child the dish, have them smell the aromas and savor the thought of eating a good meal. The French have a great saying for this: when they're feeling a little hungry close to meal-time and smell wonderful food, they say they are *mis en appétit* (which is perhaps best translated as "having one's appetite awak-ened").

I know this isn't easy. The "snack-time all the time" culture we have puts pressures on parents to let their kids snack when-ever they want, wherever they want. You're likely to encounter some resistance from your children (or their friends or other parents) when going cold turkey on random snacking. But remember: by scheduling (not forbidding) snacks, you're teach-ing your child important life lessons—and not just about food.

The Marshmallow Experiment

Could something as simple as food choices help children develop important life skills? Yes! One of the most famous (and funny) experiments to demonstrate this is the Marshmallow Experiment. The results of this experiment show how food education is a means of teaching children good habits that will stand them in good stead for life: delayed gratification and self-regulation.

In the early 1970s, Stanford professor Walter Mischel con-ducted a seemingly simple experiment.[13] One by one, the 4-year-old children whose parents had volunteered them for the experiment were invited into a small, empty room with only a chair and a desk on which had been placed a bell and a tray with two marshmallows. After each child was seated at the desk, the researcher made them an offer: either they could eat the marsh-mallow right away or they could have two marshmallows after waiting 15 minutes, while the researcher was out of the room. If they wanted the researcher to come back earlier, they could ring the bell—but then they wouldn't get the second marshmallow. Then the researcher left the room.

The hundreds of children who eventually participated in the Marshmallow Experiment were videotaped by researchers, who documented their behavior in detail. Some kids—the "low delayers"—simply popped the marshmallow into their mouths as soon as the researcher left the room. Others stared at the marshmallow for a few minutes and then rang the bell. One particularly savvy kid put the marshmallow in his mouth, but then didn't chew or swallow until time was up (although he drooled impressively!). But some kids were able to wait, usually by distracting themselves: they sang, got up and walked or danced around the room, fiddled with the bell or chair, fidgeted, or even got under the table so the marshmallow was out of sight. At the end of 15 minutes, these "high delayers" got their reward.

Mischel's team followed these children as they grew up, doing periodic surveys and interviews. Their findings were astounding. Kids who were able to delay gratification (and wait for that second marshmallow) were more likely to be successful later in life. The "high delayers" were more likely to have better S.A.T. scores (on average 210 points higher) and go further in their education. The "low delayers" had, on average, a significantly higher body-mass index and were more likely to have had problems with drugs. To some extent, these differences are innate, but Mischel also found that they related to family environment and parenting practices. Some kids didn't have the chance to practice delayed gratification as much as others. Those who did—for example, through saving up their allowance or not snacking in between meals—learned valuable life lessons that carried right through to adulthood.

Mischel also found that delayed gratification is something that most of us can learn. In later experiments, some kids were taught simple mental tricks (like pretending the marshmallow was a cloud) and were better at waiting as a result. This seems to be true in real life, too: a substantial set of kids who failed the marshmallow test went on to become successful, "high delaying" adults.

Creating an eating routine, in other words, is a great way to teach children some important life lessons. They'll be learning useful skills: moderation, self-control, and planning ahead. They'll also be learning to delay gratification and that you can make thoughtful (rather than impulsive) choices about eating. Scheduling snacks is one great way to teach these skills to children.[14]

Creating a healthy snacking routine: Getting started

If you're thinking about creating (or modifying) your family's eating routine to limit snacks, the most important thing to remember is that a routine will be positive for your child. This isn't about deprivation! It's about moderation.

You know your child best, of course. A set snacking routine won't work for some children with special needs. Children under the age of 5 (whose little tummies may need more frequent meals) may need a morning as well as afternoon snack. But the three meals plus one snack per day routine will work fine for most children 5 years of age and older. If snacking once a day is their routine, and if this routine is consistently followed, they'll adjust—probably faster than you'd believe.

You can also help your children wait longer between meals if you serve real food (rather than processed food) at both meal- and snack-time. In fact, the best way to think of snack-time is as a mini-meal. Try combinations of protein, starches, vegetables, and fruits, and avoid processed foods. Even "healthy" prepackaged food is to be avoided—it doesn't provide the same nutrients as real, fresh fruits and vegetables (and doesn't help much with table manners, either).[15]

You can also use snack-time as a great, low-pressure occasion to encourage your child to eat real (whole, unprocessed) foods. Remember: if you serve a fruit and/or vegetable at every snack (as well as every meal), your child will be much more likely to be eating their daily recommended amounts. Mealtimes will then be less of a battle. Snacks will work *for* you rather than *against* you.

What to Serve for a Satisfying, Healthy Snack?

Healthy snacks combine foods that are high in nutrients and energy-dense. Grains (carbohydrates) provide energy for busy bodies. Fruits and veggies are high in vitamins. Proteins ideally also supply a bit of healthy fats, which helps with nutrient absorption and increases the feeling of fullness (satiety), enabling your child to last until mealtime without another snack attack. Pick one item from each category for a "complete" snack. Treat snacks as a mini-meal rather than serving snacking foods, but don't be afraid to make "fun" snacks, too, such as homemade popcorn with real butter.

Fruits and Veggies	Grains	Proteins
Fresh fruit, sliced	Whole-wheat crackers	Nut butter
Sliced raw veggies (carrots, celery)	Toast	Cream cheese and/or dip for raw veggies
Fruit smoothie	Homemade popcorn with butter	Cheese
Vegetable (tomato) juice	Pita bread	Bean dip or hummus
Fruit compote (page 340)	Low- or no-sugar breakfast cereal	Milk (2% or whole)
Stewed fruit	Muffin	Luncheon meat

Most important, choose highly nutritious foods for snacks. Wean your child off juice, which is mostly empty calories (apple juice has almost as much sugar as some fizzy drinks, without much added nutritional value). Scientific studies show that children's interest in eating vegetables declines when they've had even a small amount of juice.[16]

I know this isn't easy. Dr. Jennifer Cheng, who leads the Obesity Prevention Program at Harvard University, wrote about this in the *Journal of the American Medical Association*. When counseling a patient about her overweight toddler, Dr. Cheng suggested that water be substituted for juice at snack-time. The response? Her patient, Lisa, admitted that it was hard because her toddler, Maria, threw huge tantrums if she didn't get her way. Dr. Cheng showed them the Sugar Stacks website (sugarstacks.com) and asked Lisa to help Maria count the number of sugar cubes in a container of apple juice. Lisa's jaw dropped. "Wow, that's a lot of sugar!" Dr. Cheng worked with Lisa to develop new strategies (replacing juice with chilled water, for example). To help with the transition and give Maria a sense of control, she also suggested that Lisa ask Maria if she would prefer to have one or two small frozen juice cubes or a squeeze of fresh lemon or orange in her water. As Maria continued to whine, Lisa turned to Dr. Cheng and asked, "Is this what you call tough love?" Dr. Cheng smiled back and said, "I'd just call it love."[17]

New foods at snack-time: Fun games to play

This chapter includes two games that will help your child explore new tastes so they can expand their repertoire of snack foods. Grapefruit at snack-time? Why not.

Game 9:
The Sour Fruit Game[18] (Ages 2 and up)

Main message: This game introduces your child to the idea that sour is an interesting (not necessarily bad) taste. Some of my test family kids went on to adopt grapefruit as their favorite fruit after playing this game! The point is to teach children to describe and understand the sour taste rather than just react to it. Older children will also learn that temperature changes how things taste. By playing this game, you'll encourage your child to like more "interesting" tastes so they can expand the range of foods they eat at snack-time.

My test families saw amazing results. Remember 3-year-old Lucas, who wouldn't eat a single vegetable before he started taste training? Lucas felt the same way about fruit. His mom, Jessica, told me, "Lucas would not even *lick* an orange!" However, the Sour Fruit Game had a miraculous effect on Lucas. Despite her hesitations, Jessica began by telling him that they were going to play a "fruit game." Lucas loved the idea and was very excited to get started. With a little encouragement, he picked up half an orange and started licking it, imitating his mother: "MMMMmmm ... juicy!" When Jessica told him it was sour, Lucas replied, "I *love* sour ... This is my most favorite fruit, I think!" Soon they'd moved on to grapefruit, and fruit salad became a favorite dessert. Jessica proudly reported to me, "Lucas astonished his dad by identifying the grapefruit in the fruit salad, and proceeded to tell his father— who hadn't been there for the fruit game—all about grapefruit and how much he likes it. Success!"

What you'll need:
1 pink grapefruit, peel and pith removed, sliced
1 teaspoon granulated sugar
Fruit salad that includes grapefruit (at least ½ cup per child)

What to do:
Taste test the grapefruit. Tell your child that you're going to play a fruit game, and that they'll have fun tasting different pieces of fruit. Give them two (small!) pieces of grapefruit lightly sprinkled with sugar—one straight out of the fridge and one at room temperature—and ask them to taste each piece. Now repeat the experiment, but without sprinkling the grapefruit with sugar. Ask your child to compare the different tastes and sensations. They probably liked it better with the sugar and noticed the difference between the cold and warm versions! Ask your child to describe what "sour" actually tastes like. With some kids, this may work almost too well! One of my test family moms, Teresa, reported that

her 2-year-old daughter was so excited by the discovery that she now calls grapefruit "sour" and asks for it by saying "I want sour!"

Taste test a fruit salad. Sometime later that day (or at most a few days afterward), serve your child a fresh fruit salad that includes small pieces of grapefruit. I usually recommend using fruits your child likes (such as banana, apple, and grapes). Discuss the contrasts in taste with them and explain how combining sweet with sour fruits makes both tastier. Some young kids will find it funny to make the "sour face" after eating the grapefruit—that's okay! This allows them to express their reaction to sour tastes, but not to categorize that reaction as "ew" or "yuck."

Game 10:
The Surprise Sack Game (Ages 3 and Up)

Main message: Our ideas about food depend on sight and smell as well as touch. If we can't see the food, our sense of touch can play tricks on us. This game helps kids refine their sense of touch and abilities to define textures, which is important for learning to like a broad range of foods.

In this game, a classic French taste-training technique is used to introduce an element of surprise into snack-time. It is used regularly in the French school system: kindergarteners play it in class, and teachers use it until the children are about 9 or 10 years old. Kids of all ages (and even adults) love this game because it is so surprisingly hard to guess correctly!

Safety tip: If you're playing this game with a younger child, make sure the foods you use are ones you feel are safe for your toddler to eat in case they do pop the foods in their mouth.

What you'll need:
A medium-size opaque bag (one you can't see through) with a smallish opening (a paper bag is ideal)

A variety of finger foods, including foods your child already eats as well as new foods.

Note: you don't want the bag to be too full! I recommend including no more than one or two of the following: cherry tomatoes, grapes, olives, Cheerios, Shreddies, nuts (cashews, almonds, peanuts), raisins. Think of other fun combinations—use whatever you have on hand in the kitchen!

What to do:
Hide the food items in the bag. Place your chosen food items inside the bag, *making sure your child doesn't see what you're including.*

Guess what's inside the bag! Ask your child to put their hands in the bag and to describe what they feel. Ask them to guess what is inside the bag. Then ask them to pick one thing and take it out. Repeat.

Variation for older kids: Fill two dishwashing gloves (just the fingers) with items of different textures. Loosely close the top of each glove with an elastic band so the child can't see inside but can wriggle their hand inside. Here are a few suggestions for contents:

- small rocks or gravel (smooth, hard, cold)
- bicarbonate of soda or flour (dusty, dry)
- modeling clay (soft, squishy)
- a cut-up scrubby sponge (rough, abrasive)
- a cut-up soft sponge (smooth, squishy)
- a piece of soft fabric (silky, velvety, depending on what you use)
- popcorn, couscous, barley, lentils, or small seeds you might have on hand (smooth, hard)
- sand (granular)

Ask your child to reach inside each glove and describe what they feel. Ask them to use a variety of words (more or less complex, depending on their age) to describe the different textures. Have them investigate each item by pressing on the fingers of each glove and ask them to describe what they feel when they apply pressure. After discussing the textures, ask your child to guess what is inside each finger of the glove.

The surprise sack game is akin to the many texture play games that preschools often use with children. Research suggests that younger children don't integrate visual and touch information in the same way that adults do, which is one of the reasons they can react so strongly to certain food textures.[19] Research also shows that preferences for certain textures are learned, and strongly influenced by, early exposure to a wide variety of textures.[20]

Including food in your texture play is a great way to introduce young kids to the idea that foods have different textures. If they play with dried beans today, a slippery tomato or a bumpy cucumber will become less scary tomorrow. The possibilities here are endless: you can let your children touch and play with dried rice or dried beans (but watch for choking hazards), flour, sugar, even—although not for the faint of heart—jelly!

Top Tips For Healthy Snacking

- **Set a schedule** (such as three meals and one afternoon snack per day) and then firmly and clearly explain the difference between "eating times" and "non-eating times." Note: people's eating routines may vary, and you know your child best. Three meals and two snacks per day may work for some, whereas others will be happy with one snack. The important thing is to pick a routine and stick to it.
- **Do a snack purge.** Don't carry food in your bag or car glove compartment. It will be easier for kids to accept the new schedule if they know there's no food hiding in your pockets. Try to plan your outings so that you're adhering to your schedule.
- **Be firm: don't let your child eat on demand.** If you're changing your routine, provide a simple explanation

and then stick to it. Children may whine at first if you've been providing snacks on demand. If they see that you are firm, they *will* get used to it. They'll re-adjust their eating habits accordingly so that they're eating more at meals.

- **Make sure meals are filling as well as nutritious so kids eat well and feel less hungry between mealtimes.** Most people know that a balanced, varied diet is key to good nutrition. But one equally important (but often overlooked) point is that kids need a moderate amount of healthy fats in their diet for the proper absorption of many nutrients. A small amount of fat combined with other foods will also help kids feel full for longer (bread and almond butter rather than bread and jam; full-fat yogurt or cheese alongside whole-grain crackers). Incorporating healthy fats in meals increases the "satiety" (fullness) feeling and helps kids avoid grazing and random snacking between meals.

- **Treat your snacks like mini-meals.** Eat real, whole foods that you'd be comfortable serving at a meal (such as fruits, veggies, whole grains, and proteins). Healthy, filling snacks are best. Avoid offering standard snack foods, which are often high in calories but low in nutrition—those are "treats," not food. Teach your kids the difference.

- **Choose water or milk to drink.** Sweet drinks (such as juice, soda, or sports drinks) should be treats, not regulars at snack-time. Or try making smoothies with veggies and fruit (page 320). Best of all: give your child some fruit and a glass of water.

- **Start young.** Create an eating routine that you'd like your kids to follow as adults. Unless you're dealing with specific medical issues, by the age of 5 (although in France this routine starts much earlier, by the age of 3 or 4 at the latest), children thrive on three meals and one snack per day.

Secret 4

Routines and Rituals Make Healthy Eating Automatic (and Fun!)

Nutrition-based education isn't the best way to convince kids to eat healthy foods. Instead of focusing on nutrition, the easiest way for you to get your child to eat well is to create positive rituals for *when* and *how* they eat. You know the old saying "You can lead a horse to water, but you can't make him drink"? The horse (your child) has to *want* to eat healthy foods. But nutrition-based education isn't the best way to convince them to do so. So instead of focusing on nutrition, the easiest way for you to get your child to eat well is to create positive rituals for when and how they eat. If you create good eating routines and rituals, mealtimes will work better for everyone. Your child will be more receptive to learning to eat new things, to eating healthy foods, and they will truly want to do so.

Why are routines and rituals useful? To start with, they simplify your life. They create boundaries so that you don't have to rely so much on negotiating or imposing parental authority. For example, when your child asks for a snack 20 minutes before dinner, you can gently remind them of your routine (which might be something like "no snacks 1 hour before mealtime"). Good boundaries—for example, clearly separating "times when we eat" from "times when we don't eat"—mean less stress for you.

Good boundaries also create structure in your lives. This, in turn, provides children with a sense of predictability and security, so they won't be so fussy about *when* and *what* they eat. A predictable eating hour, for example, helps them wait for dinner without snacking, even if they're feeling a bit hungry. And if vegetables and fruit are served at every meal, and no substitutes are provided, they are more likely to eat healthy offerings as a matter of course.

Most important, these routines and rituals liberate you—as a parent and as an entire family—to focus on enjoying your food and on enjoying one another's company at mealtimes. Routines (which are best understood as good habits rather than strict rules) actually mean less work and more fun for you as a parent.

I know this sounds a little hard to believe, so I'll tell you a little story about two moms—best friends—who (after reading *French Kids Eat Everything*) decided to take a summer holiday together and turn it into a food experiment. During their holiday, the two families (with five kids under the age of 10) rented cabins together and shared the cooking. They set a schedule of three meals per day and one scheduled afternoon snack. They made simple, healthy, tasty dishes that the parents were happy to eat. One meal was served for everyone—no short-order cooking. If the kids didn't want to eat what was served, they didn't have to (although they had to taste it to see if they liked it or not), but no substitutes were provided. The parents decided they wouldn't nag, cajole, chide, or even comment. Their focus was having fun; after all, it was *their* vacation, too.

At first, it was nearly all-out rebellion. The older kids were unhappy and complained, and the younger ones followed suit. But the parents held firm. "It took about a week," one of the moms later told me, "but it really worked!" Once they realized that the new approach to eating was in place, the kids came to the table and ate what was in front of them. Less time as short-order cooks meant more time for the parents to relax. They were happier at the table—and their happiness was infectious. By the end of the week, the kids were eating on a schedule and trying whatever was put in front of them. They had tried—and, to their surprise, actually liked—a few new foods. Months later, their parents are happy to report that their children are still better eaters.

So what rituals work best? Every family is different, but this chapter summarizes some rituals that have been scientifically tested and proven to work.

The "veggies (or fruits) first" ritual

Does *how* we eat influence *what* we eat? I'd never really thought about this before having children. But after having children—and struggling to figure out how to teach them to become good eaters—I slowly realized that creating good eating routines is one of the most important jobs that parents have.

Perhaps the easiest yet most amazingly effective routine I've tried is the "veggies-first" routine. *This sounds nice,* you might be thinking, *but my kids are not veggie lovers.* Well, if you adopt this approach, they just might surprise you. Researchers at the University of Pennsylvania studied the effects of serving a first course of carrots and found not only that children ate more carrots than usual, but also that they increased their vegetable consumption throughout the meal—eating more of other vegetables served later (including broccoli)![1]

Intuitively, this makes sense. If you've adopted Secret 3 (no random snacking) then your child will be feeling appropriately hungry when they get to the table, and they'll be more likely to eat more of their veggies if they're served first. Serving vegetables as a first course also makes eating vegetables automatic rather than a matter of negotiation. Because there's nothing else on the table (yet), your child won't be shuffling the veggies off to the side because something more appealing is also available, and you'll avoid the classic "No dessert if you don't eat your veggies" negotiation, which teaches kids that dinner is "yucky" and dessert is the reward. Instead, you're establishing a logical consequence: "first this, then that." Until your child has finished (or at least tried) their veggie dish (Act One), the main course (Act Two) doesn't appear on the table. This is not a punishment, by the way, but rather a logical consequence. If you have a routine in place, your child knows that their veggie plate doesn't get cleared away, and the main course isn't served, until they've eaten their veggies.

Introducing a "veggies-first" routine is harder, of course, if your child isn't a big fan of whatever is on their plate (cauliflower, anyone?). That's why teaching your child to enjoy veggies (using the taste-testing methods described in Secret 1: Kids Can *Learn* to Love Healthy Foods) is the first place to start. Once your child has a set of veggies they like, these can start appearing in the first course. In fact, the test families I worked with while writing this book—many of whose kids disliked vegetables—all found that serving veggies first made a big difference.

When Jon started his taste-training experiment, his 10-year-old son wouldn't touch most vegetables. Brandy's 2½-year-old daughter wouldn't touch any fruit except blueberries (in blueberry yogurt, that is). By the end of our three-month taste-training experiment, both were eating foods they had previously refused: Jon's son realized he loved green beans, and Brandy's daughter was eating fruit salad!

In another test family, Jessica (mom of 3-year-old Lucas) found that serving meals in courses had amazing results:

> *I've been doing "veggies first" with Lucas for the past few months. I love it! I think it's been the most effective way to get the kid to eat his veggies. I always start with a mixed green salad, cucumber salad, carrot salad, or just toss some cut-up tomatoes and other raw vegetables in a vinaigrette. He seems to love it. I don't need to prompt him to begin eating now, which is huge! I'm embarrassed to say that prior to this, he ate no vegetables ... zero. I could occasionally get him to eat a carrot stick with lunch. But now that he knows that his meals always go in a particular order, he's accepted it and digs right in. That's not to say that it was easy in the beginning. But it was amazing how little time it actually took before he began to ask, "What's my first course, Mama?"*
>
> *—Jessica*

Joy, another parent, said this about trying a meal with a "veggies-first" course:

> *We've switched to courses in our family of five (7-year-old daughter, 3-year-old daughter, 2-year-old son), and we've been skipping snacks, and they definitely eat a lot more vegetables. Serving the vegetables first, rather than American family–style of all on the table at once, has*

resulted in their eating more vegetables and less of the carbs/breads/pastas. I'm loving this, and the kids are enjoying it, too!

—Joy

If this still seems daunting, remember that kids are less likely to balk at smaller servings. Servings for kids are rarely larger than ½ cup (think small ramekin), which is a lot smaller than a lot of people think (it's about four green beans or five cherry tomatoes!). Servings are even smaller for toddlers: if your toddler is eating 2 tablespoons of vegetables three to five times per day, they're doing well! By eating these smaller portions first, children appease their hunger, and they're more likely to have a reasonable serving of the main course when it does appear on the table. Automatic portion control!

The trick is to serve these smaller servings at every meal. Smaller kids need only about 2 cups (four servings) of vegetables and fruits per day—that would be a lot to eat for any one course or at any one meal! Instead, try providing one serving of vegetables as a first course at lunch, then one serving of fruit at snack-time, and then one serving of vegetables as a first course at dinner, followed by a fresh fruit dessert. For older kids, you can progressively increase the serving sizes, as appropriate.

The most important thing about serving a meal in courses is that everyone eats the same thing—no substitutes and no short-order cooking. Kids do as we do rather than as we say; modeling good eating behaviors and healthy food preferences is one of the best way for parents to teach kids how to eat well.[2] (The wonderful thing is that this structure will help you regulate *your* eating behavior, too.) Plus, think of how much time you'll save if you're currently short-order cooking for your kids.

The casual multi-course meal ritual

Once the veggies-first method is working for you, why not introduce the multi-course meal as a family ritual? The French-style meal involves courses—as few as two courses (vegetables, then main dish) but more usually four courses (vegetables, main dish, salad and cheese, dessert). This strategy works wonders for encouraging children to eat healthy food: you separate the meal into different sections, and start with the foods you want your children to eat more of (like veggies).

Before you think this sounds like a recipe for spending your life in the kitchen, you should know that on average the French spend only 18 minutes more per day cooking than Americans do. (Just as French women manage to look impossibly elegant while spending no more time getting ready than we would take to pull on a pair of jeans. Annoying, I know.) Serving meals in courses doesn't mean spending hours preparing meals; rather, it means serving the different dishes you've prepared in a specific order.

You may be wondering, *When will my child be old enough to eat a multi-course meal?* It may be possible at a younger age than you would expect. By the time they're 5 or 6 years old, children can easily eat a three-course meal like adults, as long as the serving sizes are appropriate. Some start even younger. You know your child best—but remember, kids often surprise us with what they're willing and able to learn.

So, how do you serve a casual multi-course meal? It simply requires a little planning. Prior to inviting everyone to sit down to eat, place the things you'll need on the table: plates, cutlery, napkins, glasses, water jug, salt and pepper, a bowl of salad, a small plate of cheese, and any serving utensils you'll need. A rule of thumb: you should only have to get up from the table two or three times during dinner. As much as possible, plan in advance for everything you'll need. Make setting the table a family event— kids love helping with this. Once the table is ready, everyone sits down to eat.

Veggie starter: *About 5 minutes.* Typically, a small bowl or plate is set in front of each person at the table, with either a small serving of veggies or—in the winter—a warm, tasty soup (such as

Roasted Red Pepper and Tomato Soup, page 254). Once every-one has eaten their starter, the starter plates are cleared.

This doesn't need to be fancy! My mother-in-law sometimes simply slices an avocado in half, removes the pit, and fills the little hollowed-out space left behind with some homemade Classic Vinaigrette (page 365). The avocado (still in its skin) is eaten directly with a spoon. It's an elegant dish that takes about 30 seconds per person to prepare. *Voilà!*

Main dish: *About 10 to 15 minutes.* The main part of the meal usually consists of a protein, a starch, and a veggie side, served after the veggie starter is eaten. As the meal is casual, the pots or pans are often brought to the table and placed on trivets, and the food is served directly onto the plates so everyone can say how much (or little) they'd like.

On the weekend, when you have more time, a classic family meal might include Sweet and Sour Blueberry-Glazed Chicken (page 312), potatoes or rice, and a steamed vegetable such as green beans. Mid-week, or if you're in a rush, you might try making something simple in advance, like Ratatouille (page 258), which you can serve with couscous. The key is that everyone eats the same thing at the same time.

Salad: *About 5 to 10 minutes.* Salad is often a separate course for French (and Italian) families. You can serve it in separate bowls or on the same plate as the main course (unless the main course has a sauce or something else that would interfere with the taste of the salad). If you're truly doing this meal French-style, you'll serve the salad with cheese, which will be on a small serving plate to enable people to cut their own pieces. Usually one or two cheeses are served at most; everyone will take one small slice (about 2.5-cm square) to nibble with the salad. In many countries, such as France and Italy, people eat a salad course with most meals. This has a great effect on the kids: remember, multiple exposures to happy adults eating healthy foods increases kids' acceptance of those foods! According to one study, nearly 90 percent of French 8-year-olds like to eat lettuce. This matches my impression of kids in France: Eating salad is, for them, as normal as eating bread.[3]

Dessert: *About 5 minutes.* Fruit is a good choice for dessert; this might be as simple as a pear, kiwi, or clementine. If you'd like something fancier, you can try adding a bit of ice cream or shaved dark chocolate, but the main focus of the dessert should be fruit. For the hot lunches prepared in French schools, the rule is fresh fruit for dessert four days per week, a sweet treat on the fifth!

This might sound like a lot of work, but my test families found that it doesn't take long to settle down into the new routine. Try it once per week to start with, and treat it as a bit of a special family occasion. To make it more special, use some of the fun dinner-table activities described later in this chapter. You'll find that your child will start looking forward to your meals together, and that these are great moments in which to introduce new foods.

Negotiating "No, thank you": The "polite no" ritual

We've all seen it: a child who cringes at the sight of a particular food, covers their mouth when the food is placed on the plate, and spits it out if it's placed in their mouth. (Actually, this is a pretty accurate description of how my older daughter used to behave as a toddler.) Teaching your child to negotiate a polite "no, thank you" is a delicate art. If children are offered a food, they're allowed to decline (after tasting it, if they're following the one-bite rule). If they don't like something, the polite thing to do is say nothing, but simply leave it discreetly on the side of their plate.

There's a practical reason to teach your child how to politely say "no, thank you": scientists have found that disgust is highly contagious. Children—even infants—are very sensitive to the food likes and dislikes of the adults around them.[4] Basic rules of politeness about negative reactions to food will enable you to limit food dislikes spreading from one sibling to another.

Remember: refusing food is a great way to get attention—lots of it. The challenge for you is *not* to give your child attention for being picky. Give them attention when they're eating well. The behaviors you focus on are the ones that will grow.

Of course, parent-led modeling is powerful, but it can only go so far. Anyone with school-age children knows that peers have a powerful influence on children's food likes and dislikes. In fact, preschoolers are similar: even little children will be more likely to eat a food (or reject it) based on what other children are saying and doing.

One powerful experiment demonstrated peer influences on food preferences. British researchers decided to test the peer effect amongst young children.[5] They created two "new" target foods that the children (between the ages of 5 and 7) were unlikely to have experienced before: potato bread and quorn, which were colored blue and given the names "fodrick" and "gwark." The new (and admittedly fearsome-sounding) foods were given to the children on paper plates, together with other snack foods (grapes, cheese, bread, and carrots).

The paper plates were presented to the children as part of a special activity day in which older children (8- to 11-year-olds from another school) were visiting the classroom. Unbeknownst to the younger children, these older peers were part of the experiment: they'd been trained by the researchers to encourage (or discourage) the younger children to eat the new foods. Praising the "fodrick" and "gwark" with lines rehearsed in advance, half of the older children ate the blue foods with gusto at snacktime. The preschoolers at their tables followed suit. The other half of the confederates refused to touch the food and made negative comments; children at their tables avoided the "gwark" and "fodrick" as if they were radioactive (and who could blame them)? What's even more impressive is that the children who did try the blue foods were more likely to try other new foods in the weeks following the experiment—even without extra encouragement!

This suggests a simple ritual at mealtimes: inviting each child to say something positive about the meal. Negative comments can be kept to oneself; it's helpful to remind children that the polite thing to do when confronted with a food one doesn't like is to simply say nothing (or at least not to make a big deal of it). It's important to respect the feelings and efforts of the person who made the meal.

You might even try some positive peer pressure of your own if you know a child (often older) who can act as a role model. If you don't have cousins or neighbors' kids handy, try to find a willing babysitter on your next night out. Instead of serving your kids pizza, try serving something adventurous that you know your babysitter likes. Or you might try finding an older child of a friend who might be a bit picky but would relish the opportunity to help positively influence your child. The older child might, in turn, be tempted to be more adventurous themselves—an unexpected benefit to his parents!

Online peers work well, too, such as the "Food Dudes" program (fooddudes.co.uk), which offers rewards to kids who eat the "Life Force" foods (fruit and vegetables) favored by its superhero characters, battling with the evil Junk Punks who are attempting to steal energy from children all over the world.[6] (This cleverly uses "magical thinking": the qualities we associate with certain foods are often attached to the personality and character of those who consume them.[7])

The table talk ritual

At our house, we've recently started asking each family member to tell a story about the day. Cornell Professor Brian Wansink advocates keeping children at the table and taking the attention off the food (and power struggles at bay) through the use of distraction. Each member of the Wansink family answers four questions: What was the high point of the day? What was the low point? Whom did he or she most appreciate? What direction is your compass pointing tomorrow? (See Game 12: The Rose, Thorn, and Bud Game for a similar strategy.) It's okay to talk about the food, of course, but it shouldn't become the focal point of the meal. (Note: table talk is greatly aided by banning electronic devices of any kind at the table. This means you as well as your kids!)

Fun family conversations may have another unexpected benefit: getting kids to stay longer at the table. Make sure kids are comfortably seated; for example, toddlers need foot support even after they outgrow a high chair. Try buying special kid-size cutlery for them, and asking them to set the table themselves. Tell jokes, tell stories, or simply chat! Parents are often at their most animated (and kids often enthralled) at the dinner table in countries where families prioritize mealtimes (think of every Italian family dinner you've ever seen in a movie).[8] If you start telling some of your funniest or most interesting stories, your kids might surprise you with their sudden interest in being at the table.

"Happy meal" rituals

Special, celebratory meals are found in every culture. Births, deaths, religious celebrations, and historic events are all associated with special foods. Why not create your own meal rituals for special occasions? They create great family memories. Françoise, from one of my test families, sent in this anecdote:

> *One of my best friends has a great family tradition. On each person's birthday every year they have a family meal (the friends celebrate another day). The kids decide on the full menu and then write it out. The parents prepare all their wished-for dishes. The only rules are that the menus have to be different every year and include a good variety of foods. So the kids really feel in control and creative. Also, they decorate the birthday girl's or boy's place setting with a crown of flowers and a little vase with a bouquet. And the child or even adolescent sits at the head*

*of the table! Now that her children are grown up (19 and
21), they all remember those times around the table as
some of the best times of their childhood.*

—Françoise

Other test families shared their experiences of creating everyday
family food rules that made each meal special and more enjoyable.
Below is a list of some of the rules I collected from my test families.
Some of these were drafted by children, as you can tell!

One other point: Too many rules all at once, or draconian
enforcement, won't help your cause. The family table should be
a place where you recharge your batteries and are positive with
your kids, not a source of stress. Feel free to pick and choose the
rules that might best suit your family, and remember: this list is
aspirational.

- Wait to start eating until everyone has been served
  (my godmother calls this the "Royal Fork" rule—the
  kids love watching her, waiting to see when she raises
  her fork to her mouth, before they start to eat!).
- Put the napkin in your lap and use it to wipe your
  mouth and fingertips (only).
- Every child should use cutlery according to his or her
  abilities (babies will be learning about spoons; toddlers about forks; school-age children about knives
  and forks, and which cutlery choices to make for different dishes).
- Comment nicely on the foods you like (and say nothing about the foods you don't like).
- Have a "nice eating face"—no noises, no slurping, no
  bites bigger than can fit in your mouth, chew with
  your mouth closed, the utensil goes in with a bite-size
  piece and comes out empty.
- Only polite requests for second helpings will be met
  (a logical consequence that keeps things positive but
  firmly polite).

- Adults must also be on their best behavior: no lectures and no complaining about the cooking or the food served.
- Children must wait until everyone has finished their main course before they can ask to be excused. (Younger children may asked to be excused when they are done, but once they are excused they can't come back to the table for more food.)

Some families write these rules down and stick them on the fridge as a reminder. If you make a list, involve your child from the outset—they'll take more ownership of these ideas if you do. Most important: don't get too hung up on policing perfect manners. Praising good behavior at the table will work better in the long run than commenting on bad behavior. The basic rules of politeness are meant to enable you to enjoy the meal together and to teach your child to be considerate of others at the table. Keep this goal your focus and keep your cool (no easy task, I know), and your child will eventually follow your routines. This might seem hard at first, but it will save you stress in the long term. As your child gets the hang of these new routines, they'll come to expect them—and even feel proud when they can help keep everyone on track.

Of course, whatever ritual you choose should be one that is fun for your family. Aim to make mealtime one of the most fun, relaxing moments that the family spends together. The two games below are designed to help you do just that.

Game 11:
The Smiley Face Game (Ages 1 and Up)

Main message: This is one of the simplest games in this book and also one of the most effective. My test families were often amazed that even older children responded well to smiley faces on plates, in soups, and so on. Don't do this every day (or the effect wears off fast), but once in a while is a great reminder that food is fun. For younger kids, making a simple happy face part of their regular meal routine sets the right tone for eating healthy food in a fun atmosphere.

There are many variations on this game, but here's a simple example of a smiley face veggie plate that you can serve at snacktime or as the first course at dinnertime. Of course, you can invent your own options—or let the kids compose their smiley faces themselves!

What you'll need (per smiley face):
3 or 4 cherry tomatoes
2 lettuce leaves
1 baby carrot
2 smallish cucumber slices

For the mouth: Cut the cherry tomatoes in half and lay them side-by-side in a semi-circle.

For the hair: Slice the lettuce into thin strips and mound it at the top of the plate.

For the nose: Slice the tip off the baby carrot (for a long nose!) or chop it in half and place it in the center of the face.

For the eyes: Use cucumber slices, cut as you like, and arrange them side-by-side.

Kids also love a "melting" smiley face as a garnish for soups and purées. Use little dabs of butter (or another soup or a garnish or purée of a contrasting color) to make eyes, nose, a mouth, and hair. Watch as your child eats up the smiley face—hurry up before it disappears!

Game 12:
The Rose, Thorn, and Bud Game (Ages 5 and Up)

Main message: Family mealtime is a time for sharing stories about the day. Your kids will eat better (and find it easier to sit still for longer at the table) if you have interesting conversations to keep them entertained.

The Rose, Thorn, and Bud game is one of our family favorites. Each person in the family takes a turn to tell everyone else about their day, answering three questions: "What was your rose?" (a good thing that happened today), "What was your thorn?" (a bad thing that happened), and "What is your rosebud?" (something they're looking forward to). This simple ritual avoids the conversational dead-end of "how was your day?" ("*Fine.*") and helps them appreciate that life is made up of good and bad moments—roses don't come without thorns, and there's always something to look forward to. Many families make this game a part of their daily dinner ritual.

Top Tips for Making Healthy Eating Automatic and Fun

- **Serve veggies first, at lunch, dinner, and snack-time.** You'll find that your child will automatically start eating and enjoying them more.
- **Use peer pressure positively!** Praise your child when they try something new or learn to like something new. Teach your child to *politely* say "no, thank you"—without criticizing the food—so that food refusals don't affect others at the table.
- **Use table talk to keep your child interested and motivated.** They'll sit longer at the table and be more motivated to join you at mealtimes. Ask questions and tell stories.

- **Use family food rules.** Rules will keep everyone on track and mealtimes happy rather than harried.
- **Adopt a motto.** "One family, one meal!" (Or my personal favorite: "I offer two choices at mealtime. Take it, or leave it!")
- **Create special family meal traditions.** Whether once a week or once a year, your child will associate special meals with special family memories.

Secret 5

Kids Don't Need Kids' Food

Is variety the spice of life? The Japanese (one of the longest-lived, least-obese nations on the planet) think so. Japanese tradition emphasizes the importance of a varied diet. Government guidelines advise both children and adults to eat 30 different foods per day and 100 different foods per week![1] Children learn these magic numbers in nutrition classes at school. A traditional school lunch in Japan would include steamed rice with at least two fresh vegetables, fish, and fruits—a far cry from some of our standards (pizza for breakfast, anyone?).

One of the tragic ironies of the modern, industrialized food system (which is very good at distributing large quantities of food) is that the variety of foods we eat has declined despite the ever-increasing number of apparent choices available. Many kids eat a relatively small range of foods. For example, half of the vegetables consumed by children in the United States are potatoes—in the form of french fries. For many children, "kids' food" constitutes the bulk of their diet.

Is "kid-friendly" food addictive?

Is kids' food a sort of "gateway drug" to an over-reliance on processed food as a teen and adult? Sociologist and family food counselor Dr. Dina Rose thinks so. She argues that the high concentration of salt, sugar, and fat in many processed foods targeted at children makes them more likely to crave processed food as adults.[2] These cravings may intensify over time. In a recent study of kids' ice-cream eating habits, researchers found that kids who regularly eat ice cream need to eat larger quantities to get the same sense of satisfaction (which was called a "high" in the ensuing media coverage).[3] Former FDA commissioner David Kessler even argues that eating foods loaded with fat, salt, and sugar (particularly in the optimized combinations that the food industry uses) actually changes the chemistry of our brains, literally creating the conditions for addiction to fast food.[4] Children, he argues, are particularly at risk: they have the most "plastic" (responsive) and thus vulnerable brain chemistries, and eating fast food young can literally hard-wire them to be fast food customers for life.[5]

Dr. Rose summed it up best in her post on the *Psychology Today* website, where she argued that so-called "child-friendly" foods are addictive in the same way as drugs.[6] She points to the fact that the vast majority of these foods are designed to give a flavor "hit" that unprocessed foods can't match. Kids get addicted to this "flavor hit" and come back for more. Once they're hooked, it's hard to wean them off—as any parent who has tried to do so knows. Marketers know this, too: in the US, while traditional broccoli and corn producers are seeing slumps in sales, new genetically modified innovations such as Finest Supersweet Broccoli and Sunshine Sweet Corn are hitting the shelves, designed to cater to our growing habituation to sweet tastes.[7]

Why is this a problem? Experts argue that giving mostly bland foods to babies tends to produce kids with limited taste preferences. As a result, some kids get "stuck" with a limited range of flavors and tend to prefer bland tastes and simple textures. For example, babies reared on white rice cereal are more likely to crave white bread.

Parents fall into the habit of feeding "kid-friendly" foods to their children for many reasons. We might assume that pickiness is a permanent part of our kids' personality, rather than a temporary phase, so we don't gently persist and help them get over it. Or we're busy, and it's just easier to serve the kids the same foods over and over again. Chances are that you know at least one child who doesn't eat any fruit or vegetables. Many more children subsist on a "beige food" diet consisting of white bread, pasta, and processed cereals (and I fully admit that this was my girls' diet when they were little, before our experiences in France opened my eyes). As discussed in Secret 2: Marketing Healthy Food to Your Kids Really Works!, the result is a food literacy deficit: our children know less and less about food, and are willing to eat fewer and fewer things, raising the risk of micronutrient deficiencies, obesity, and associated health problems. This is an issue for families across the socio-economic spectrum: under-nutrition (not enough food) remains a serious concern, even in wealthy countries, but malnutrition (not enough nutritious food) is also an issue.

It's not all bad news, though! Children who are exposed to more variety will have an easier time following a healthier diet; "taste training" has hard-wired their brains to be more receptive to doing so. This is true for adults as well: the Iowa Women's Health Study (designed to test the effects of healthy eating on breast cancer) found that women who started a healthy "real food" diet eventually developed aversions to the fast and processed foods they used to like.[8] Kids *can* be weaned from "kids' food," as Jon, a dad in my test family group, found out:

We had tried serving 8-year-old Sarah "real" chicken before, but she was always resistant. We used to take that to mean she was a born picky eater and would offer her something else for dinner. She loves breaded nuggets and used to have them two or three times a week. We used to buy big bags of them at the grocery store and keep them in the freezer, but don't do so any longer, so they are not an option for her. The other night, we made the Sweet and Sour Blueberry-Glazed Chicken [page 312], and I just served it up and mentioned how very sweet it was. Her 15-year-old brother didn't get a chance to say anything before Sarah scraped off the blueberries and quickly tried a small piece and commented that it was sweet. She then proceeded to finish that piece and ask for another, which she also ate. All without much discussion regarding the food! My wife and I gave each other the "don't say anything" look, as we didn't want to do anything to derail the success. Our son had a second helping, too. This was a first for Sarah—who had always refused to eat non-nugget chicken. It was a real breakthrough!

—Jon

Jon's story contains many lessons: if you serve food in appetizing ways, even the pickiest eaters may learn to like it; even young children can enjoy supposedly "adult" tastes; and perhaps the most important lesson of all, adults and kids should eat the same thing—mostly "real" food. Kids simply won't eat healthy foods unless you increase the supply of the healthy foods and reduce the availability of junk and fast food. The bonus is that eventually they'll start preferring (and even asking for) healthier foods. This has several advantages:

- **It's less work.** You'll be making one meal for the whole family (avoiding short-order cooking).
- **It's cheaper.** Do the math on homemade oatmeal versus those instant sachets and you'll see what I mean. If you don't believe me, visit the amazing "100 Days of Real Food" blog (100daysofrealfood.com), which tells the story of a family of four living on unprocessed, "real" foods for 100 days—all for less than the average family food budget.
- **Your kids will eat better (and so will you).** Kids are natural mimics, and they'll copy what mom or dad does. If dad eats salad while sitting at the table, Fred will likely do the same. If dad gobbles cookies from the packet while standing in the kitchen, guess what?

The wonderful secret weapon of this "real food" approach is the fact that kids' flavor preferences can also be trained to dislike fake food. Our daughters' friend Antoine—the son of French friends of ours who moved to Vancouver—is a good example. At the age of 3, Antoine refused to eat the store-bought, edible-oil-product-laced cakes served at the birthday parties of his new friends. "It doesn't taste good," was his response (and in my opinion, he was right). His mother proudly told me the story, affirmed by the fact that her at-home taste training had already enabled Antoine to detect—and dislike—the taste of mass-produced fake food.

Now, you may be wondering what "real food" is! There are a million experts out there who will advise you on different diets, approaches, and gimmicks. I like Michael Pollan's definition: "Don't eat anything your grandmother wouldn't recognize as food." That means string cheese is out, cheddar is in. (There are more examples at the end of this chapter.)

A "real food" approach suggests that we limit the quantities of highly processed foods (such as sugar) that kids love. This is obviously important for our health, but it's also a question of taste. Lori, one of my test family moms, used this explanation with her kids:

> *I told our two girls that sugar is like a black crayon in a picture. A little can be really neat. But if you colored a beautiful picture and then colored over all of it with black, you couldn't see any of it. That's what sugar does to a dish: a little is neat. A lot hides all of the other flavors. Eat a lot of it all the time, and your tongue can't taste anything other than sugar. It makes for a super boring life. I love the fact that this explanation isn't about sugar being bad for you, but rather that it makes for a boring, monotone taste. It's so true. And I think that kids really understand these taste-based explanations.*
>
> *—Lori*

Weaning your family from kids' food: Do a family food inventory

An inventory is a great way to get started on reforming your family's eating habits. Start by making a list of the kids' foods you have in your house. For each item, write down a "real food" equivalent. Hint: if you can't think of a real food equivalent, it's perhaps wise to think of crossing that item off your shopping list altogether. Next time you go shopping, try mostly buying from the real food category and limit the rest. It's important to limit, rather than forbid, kids' food, because you don't want this to backfire with a forbidden fruit effect in which your child develops preferences for the very things they're denied.[9] The best strategy is to divert your child's attention (by always having tasty fresh fruit on hand, for example), rather than appearing to police their eating habits.

I know that this sounds challenging. Think of it this way: in traditional food cultures there is no "kids' food." Kids eat what adults eat, and they do so at a young age; often as soon as they can chew or be reliably trusted to maneuver a spoon somewhere close to the vicinity of their mouths. Kids are hardwired to be able to eat this way; they're more than capable of doing so.

When making your list of things to eat (and things to limit), remember: kids do as we do, rather than as we say. If you're eating lots of fruits and veggies, your children are more likely to as well. If you honestly enjoy them, you're increasing the chances they will as well. If you're trying new foods with enthusiasm, they're more likely to take a bite. Explaining why kids need to eat healthy foods helps (and certainly nutritional information can't hurt, in moderation), but most kids will learn best through consistent parental role modeling.[10]

Sample Food Inventory

Kids' Food Item	Real Food Alternative
Sugary breakfast cereals	Slow-cook oatmeal (not instant)
White bread	Multigrain or whole-wheat bread
Artifically sweetened yogurt	Plain yogurt with a small amount of jam
Juice drinks	Homemade smoothies or lemonade (page 327)
Fruit leather	Fresh fruit
Frozen fish sticks	Fresh fish
Cheese strings	Cubes or slices of Cheddar cheese
Breakfast bars	Crunchy granola (try it with a bit of honey drizzled on top)

Weaning your child off kids' food will take time, but it's worth it. Essentially, you're reverse engineering the taste-training process, weaning your child from unhealthy to healthy tastes. Think of it like rehab for your child's taste buds! Once you have done your family food inventory and brought some new options into your pantry, there are three different approaches that you can mix and match: gradual substitution, the "one new thing per day" rule, and the "rotation" rule.

Gradual substitution

You can now start gradually substituting real food items in your diet. Note: the following combinations are meant to allow you to transition your child toward healthier foods; over time, aim to reduce the processed ingredients.

- Switch from white bread to sourdough, and then to multigrain.

- Try making a half-and-half pasta sauce—half store-bought, half homemade. Over time increase the proportion of homemade sauce until you eliminate the store-bought sauce altogether.
- Mix whole-grain pasta with regular pasta, and whole-grain (brown) rice with white rice.
- Serve healthy breakfast cereals (for example, slow-cook oatmeal) and use the processed kind as a sort of topping.

We recently rotated through different kinds of oatmeal, convincing our kids that rolled oats were edible and then weaning them off the instant variety. Now they don't even ask for the instant kind any more. They had it recently at a friend's house and noticed it didn't seem as satisfying or tasty. Success!

Here are some suggestions for specific goals that you might choose for your family.

- **Eat mostly 100 percent whole grains** (such as 100 percent whole-wheat bread, not white bread; ditto for cereals).
- **Make veggies and fruits half your diet.** Remember, half of our adult food consumption should be fruits and veggies, so your child should be working toward that goal. Serving veggies and fruits *first* at every meal is a simple way to help your child learn this proportion rule over time.
- **Eat healthy fats and avoid fake fats.** Don't consume high-fructose corn syrup (no sugary kids' cereals, no soft drinks, no fake icing—it's in a lot of stuff!) or anything made with hydrogenated oils and trans fats. Note: unprocessed fat (such as olive oil or butter) is not only okay in moderation, it's necessary! Kids need it for their development, and some vitamins are fat-soluble. Plus a little fat in a meal increases your feeling of fullness and helps you last longer between

meals. Harvard Medical School researchers have found that eating moderate amounts of healthy fat is a good strategy for losing weight and keeping it off.[11]

- **Everything in moderation.** A little unprocessed fat is okay, such as olive oil or butter. A little salt is okay. A little chocolate is definitely okay. You get the point!

- **Teach your child the difference between food (which we eat often) and treats (which we eat once in a while).** At your meals, and at snack-time, eat food. Treats— including candy, cake, cookies, french fries, and cola—are once-in-a-while treats. For example, we have potato chips at parties and whenever we have people over, but otherwise they're not in the house. This also helps avoid labeling foods "good" or "bad," which you shouldn't do, as it sets up emotional associations (like guilt) for your child and can lead to disordered eating.

- **Make sure your child gets enough water.** Juice is for special occasions. If your child wants fruit juice or soda, encourage them to eat fruit instead.

- **Substitute homemade treats for junk food.** Good options include plain yogurt with a spoonful of fruit compote, juice and fruit popsicles, small amounts of good-quality chocolate, fresh and dried fruits, home-made popcorn, homemade cakes.

The rotation rule

Now that your child is starting to eat healthy versions of their favorite foods, it's time to introduce a little more variety into their diet. This doesn't mean going overboard. Kids have their favorites (just like adults), and their individual taste preferences should be respected.

Many adults do tend to vary their meals. If you ate pasta for dinner last night, you're less likely to want it again the next night. However, it's easy to get into a rut of feeding your child the same thing over and over again if they accept very few foods. You can start to introduce variety by rotating your approach to making the dishes your child likes to eat. For example, if your child likes cheese on pasta, serve shredded Cheddar one day and grated Parmesan the next. Or if they like raw carrots, try serving them cooked. Use the flavors they like to introduce them to new flavors (the friendly flavor technique discussed in Secret 1: Kids Can *Learn* to Love Healthy Foods). Your child is never too young to start getting more variety in their food (although with babies less than a year old, you should wait a day or so after introducing a new food to see if it is tolerated well).

More variety has psychological benefits: kids don't get stuck in liking foods or dishes prepared a specific way. They learn to expect novelty—and to enjoy it! My French sister-in-law even deliberately varied the heat of the formula in the bottles she gave to her babies so that they wouldn't get used to demanding it at one specific temperature. (Well, she did that deliberately with the first one, but it was a "that's life" parenting survival strategy by the time the second baby arrived.) You can also model this strategy for your child when you make everyday choices: "I had an apple at lunch, so I'll have an orange now." Variety makes things fun, and if food is less boring, kids will be more engaged.

The "something new every day" rule

Introducing something new works best at a relaxed family meal—preferably in the evenings, when you have time to talk about the food and aren't pressuring your child to eat because you have to run out the door. If you can't manage a sit-down family meal in the evenings, try leaving a little more time in the mornings for a more relaxed breakfast. Variety can appear at breakfast, too: you can serve different types of fruits, make new flavors of homemade smoothies, or serve different types of cereals.

The taste-testing strategies explored on page 33 will be helpful here, too, if you aren't already trying them. Remember: it's normal to have food preferences. We all do. Individual taste differences are real and to some degree innate. However, this doesn't mean that kids can't learn to like new foods. If you make tasting a new food once per day (or per week) part of your routine, your child is more likely to be cooperative.

Increasing variety: Keep it positive

When introduced to something new, children often respond "no" to the question "Do you like this food?" But how can they dislike it if they don't know it? What they really mean is that they're not familiar with it. It's your job to expose them to the new food, in as gentle and fun a manner as possible. (See the simple taste test ideas on page 33.) One of the best ways to help kids be eager about trying new dishes is to familiarize them first. Think of it as helping your child to get to know new people (each person has their own distinctive personality). Help your child warm up by introducing them to foods as if they were new and interesting characters in their lives. Let younger kids "meet" their veggies in raw form first. Toddlers can help wash them. Older kids can help cook them! Doing this regularly—and, for more selective eaters, *before* you ask them to eat these foods—helps kids get over their reluctance. Sometimes this means being creative about recipes, as Roberta, one of my test family moms, explains:

> *If there's a food one of my kids doesn't like very much, such as eggplant, I try to serve it in different ways. This gives me a better chance of landing on a recipe that they actually like. Also, if they say "I don't like eggplant," then I can respond, "But you've never tasted it this way. I think this is the dish that will make eggplant your most favorite food!" This usually piques their curiosity, and they always try at least a few bites. Switching up cooking techniques also gets them to eat the food a few more times, so eventually they simply get used to the flavor. I've seen this work beautifully with my 7-year-old, who now eats all the foods he "hated" three years ago, including eggplant.*
>
> —Roberta

Think about what your child ate for lunch this week. In Japan (where children deftly handle chopsticks by the time they're in preschool), children eat fish and rice on a daily basis. In Peru, they eat quinoa porridge. In China, they might eat bok choy seasoned with hot peppers, or spicy noodle soup. In France, dishes like radish salad, roasted fish, and cauliflower casserole regularly show up on school lunch menus. As astounding as it may sound, kids actually *eat* this stuff. The reason is simple: they've learned to like it. In fact, they've been taught to like it—by parents and extended families, friends and peers, and teachers.

Some cultures are better at exposing their kids to vegetables than others, and at encouraging children to develop a broad set of food "likes." Chinese parents (and schools) have traditionally demanded a respectful attitude; adults disapprove of children expressing an aversion to individual dishes.[12] In France, expressing dislike of any dish on the table is viewed as a serious breach of manners.

Remember, children increase their liking of vegetables, and their consumption of vegetables, if they are asked to taste them regularly (not just look, but *actually taste*).[13] This effect is heightened if a greater variety of fruits and vegetables is present at home.[14] This even works on babies: one study found that infants who were given a different vegetable every day for a week were more likely to eat yet another veggie—green beans, in this case—when it was offered.[15]

French parents and schools typically adopt a "maximum variety" approach, and so French children have an expectation of novelty. Schools aren't allowed to serve the same dish more than once per month, and even provide suggested dinner menus to parents to help them simplify the task of not repeating anything on that week's lunch menu. "We had chicken on Monday, so let's have fish today" would be a typical reflection from a parent. Contrast this with the North American approach, where the same foods—tasting exactly the same way—are served day in and day out. This increases the likelihood of kids having narrow, rigid food preferences.

Variety, naturally: (Re)Discover seasonal foods

A simple way to maximize variety and exposure to new foods is to simply follow the seasons. With each season, new foods are available. This used to happen naturally: children got to know a variety of foods because they spent more time with adults preparing foods as well as planting, cultivating, and harvesting them. My uncles and aunts, growing up in a large farming family, still talk about the fresh taste of the first ears of summer corn, the excitement when the year's first berries were ripe, and the flavor of home-grown tomatoes.

I don't want to romanticize this kind of life or minimize the backbreaking work that still goes with it in many parts of the world. My relatives also remember the sheer exhaustion of round-the-clock work in harvest season, worrying about the weather, and the missed opportunities as kids were pulled from school at a young age to help out on the farm. Nor was their diet especially diverse (an orange was a once-a-year treat at Christmas). But the fact remains that the modern food system—with its convenience and global reach—has broken the links between seasonality and family meals, and enabled us to cater to (and even foster) kids' limited food repertoires.

Think I'm exaggerating? A recent article in the journal *Appetite* shows that parents don't expose children to foods that the parents themselves don't like, which may make picky eating worse. Why? Because this will reduce acceptance of those foods in the long-term, and negatively affect what scientists call "flavor learning." Researchers concluded, "To promote variety in children's diets, parents should model healthy behaviors by actively introducing new and previously disliked foods to their own and their child's diet, even if they themselves do not like these foods."[16] The researchers picked vegetables that don't tend to be on the list of kids' favorites: Brussels sprouts, eggplant, and cabbage.

Read that list over again: Brussels sprouts. Eggplants. Cabbage. Do *you* like these vegetables? How did *you* react when you read them? Chances are you didn't like at least one of them. Now think of other vegetables you don't like. How many of those have you offered to your child?

My "vegetable I love to hate" was always cauliflower—I would never buy it, and was always surprised to see anyone eating it—but I figured out a cauliflower recipe I enjoy eating (Cauliflower Gratin, page 232). When my kids saw me learning to enjoy cauliflower, they followed suit. One child is more enthusiastic than the other, but both will eat it, and it's now one of our family's preferred vegetables.

Our taste-training experiments have surprised even me sometimes! My 5-year-old daughter, Claire, is a good example of this. The other day she was dipping some veggies in homemade hummus with me. By accident, she got a small piece of raw garlic (I guess I hadn't quite blended it properly). "Ouch!" she cried, sticking out her tongue and spitting the little sliver of garlic on her plate, eyeing it suspiciously. "Drink some water," I said. But instead, she reached out and popped a piece of cut-up tomato in her mouth. My husband and I said nothing, as we know better than to comment too much when the kids undertake a food experiment. "It was stinging, but the tomato makes it taste better," she said, wonderingly. And then she ate another piece of tomato. (Mexican kids apparently go through a similar process when they start to learn to eat hot sauce with every meal, at about the same age.)

Just to be clear: the goal of this book is not to get your child to enjoy raw garlic—I'm not even sure that Claire will be a garlic lover. The goal is to have children be open to trying new foods and appreciating food sensations—even apparently unpleasant ones.

Before you get started, remember the most important point about taste training: you need to believe that your kids *can* and *will* eat everything. Don't assume they won't like strong tastes or flavors, or things that you don't like. Explore the tastes together as if you were on a fun family food adventure.

Fun games for introducing your child to more variety

Using the three fun games below, you can help expose your child to variety in texture and color, and help them understand how "artificial" variety might be produced through food coloring. These games are particularly fun, as they all involve "fooling" your taste buds. (The recipes that start on page 211 are designed to foster a varied diet, as they present four different ways of eating common vegetables and fruits.)

Game 13:
Terrific Textures (Ages 3 and Up)

Main message: Children often resist new foods because the foods feel strange in their mouths. This game introduces your child to a range of textures and enables them to develop a vocabulary for describing them. It will also help them learn to appreciate different "mouth sensations" without the pressure to eat they might feel at the dinner table.

Make sure to do this experiment when your child is somewhat (but not too) hungry and explain that it is a "taste experiment" or a "fun tasting game." Make it fun!

What you'll need: Choose two foods—one your child likes (the "I like it" food), and one they're learning to like (the "learning to like" food). The key is to vary the textures. For example, if your child likes apples, you would prepare (for each person participating in the game):

1 slice of fresh apple *(crunchy)*
1 small glass of apple juice *(juicy)*
1 dried apple *(chewy)* (you can make these by baking apple slices at 180°C/gas 4 for 30 minutes)
1 apple chip *(crispy)* (leave the dried apple slices in the

oven for another 20 minutes, or until they totally dry
out)

1 spoonful of applesauce *(soft)*

1 small piece of apple peel, preferably unwaxed and
organic *(smooth)*

Do the same for the "learning to like" food. For example,
if your child is learning to like tomatoes:

1 slice of un-ripe (green) tomato *(firm)*

1 slice of ripe tomato *(soft)*

1 small glass of tomato juice *(juicy)*

1 sun-dried tomato *(chewy)*

1 spoonful of tomato sauce *(soft)*

If your child doesn't like apples, try to think of another food that
could be prepared with multiple textures. For some kids, this
might mean using a soggy (soft) versus a dry (crunchy) Cheerio.
Potatoes might also fit the bill (raw potato, potato chip, boiled
potato, french fry). As long as it's a food your child likes that can
be varied in texture, you can adapt it to this experiment.

What to do:
Taste test the "I like it" food. One by one, taste each sample.
Discuss which words you would use to describe each texture.
Ask your child to describe other foods with similar textures,
including ones that they don't like. Encourage your child to think
of these as "foods I am learning to like" rather than "foods I
dislike."

Describe the textures. Ask your child to identify the textures they
like. Then ask them to identify textures they don't like.

Taste test the "learning to like it" food. Follow the steps above:
One by one, taste each sample. Discuss what words you would
use to describe each texture. Ask your child to describe other
foods with similar textures, including ones that they don't like.

Describe the textures. Ask your child to describe the textures using as many words as they can. Make sure to try each sample yourself and comment on the different textures. In many cases, your child's natural curiosity will stimulate them to give the food a taste (or maybe just a lick at first). Be patient!

You can also use texture to add a bit of fun to your meals. For example, when my younger daughter (then a preschooler) was being picky about raw carrots, I bought a bag of baby carrots and cooked half (immersed in boiling water so they would stay bright orange), leaving the other half raw. I then put them on a plate on the table at snack-time, with a few cooked and raw carrots intermingled. I offered them to my husband as well as my older daughter. We had a great time guessing whether our carrots would make a loud crunch or be silent. After seeing us laughing for a few minutes with the "carrot crunch game," my younger daughter joined in. She delighted in making the loudest "crunch" of all!

Variation: Fooling Your Taste Buds
Older kids will have fun with this version of the Terrific Textures game.

What you'll need:
1 crunchy potato
1 crunchy apple
1 blindfold

What to do: Prior to beginning the game, and *without your child watching*, peel and thinly slice the potato and apple, making sure that your slices are as identical in size as possible. Cover them up, then invite your child to play the game.

First, have your child sit down and then blindfold them. Second, ask them to plug their nose tightly. Let them know they are going to get something to eat, and place a slice of either potato or apple in their hands.

Ask your child to bite into it and identify what it is. Then place the other slice into their hand, again asking them to taste and identify it. Ask "was that the same food, or two different foods?" Most children will have difficulty distinguishing one from the other because the textures of apple and potato are similar and holding your nose makes flavors difficult to taste. Older kids will love to play this game on an unsuspecting adult.

Variation: Texture Play

A variation on this game involves texture play.[17] If you have younger children, you might want to start off with this approach. The main purpose of texture play is to give children a sensory experience about texture. Texture plays an important role in how food actually tastes and affects our perceptions about how filling a food is.[18] Texture play gives children more confidence about different textures, and more ideas—and vocabulary—about the relationship between texture and taste. Here are some of my favorite items to play with:

- bicarbonate of soda and water (makes a gooey texture when squeezed)
- large dried beans (such as kidney beans)
- rice
- sand
- small dried beans or pulses (such as lentils)

Place each item in a separate cup and set the cups on a surface onto which your child can pour, stir, and manipulate the foods, then step back and let them play!

If your child is interested, you can also try manipulating the texture of foods with heat. For example, experiment with the texture (and taste and color) of peanut butter by heating or cooling it (or roasting it).

Older kids might be interested in learning about additives that change the texture of foods, such as guar gum or xanthan gum. Next time you're at the supermarket, ask your child to read some labels for these additives.

Game 14:
The Color Confusion Experiment (Ages 6 and up)

The main message: This simple experiment teaches kids how color can influence their sense of taste (that's why processed foods often use artificial colors to increase visual appeal). This experiment also teaches your child to be wary of how their senses can be fooled through the use of artificial colors.

What you'll need:
5 identical glasses (clear glass or plastic)
Water
5 tablespoons granulated sugar
Red food coloring

What to do:
Prepare the experiment. Without your child being able to see what you're doing, pour ½ cup of water in each glass then add 1 tablespoon of sugar to each glass, mixing until dissolved. Now add red food coloring to each glass: 1 drop in the first glass, 2 drops in the second glass, 3 drops in the third glass, 4 drops in the fourth glass, and 5 drops in the fifth glass. The result should be a range of colors: from light pink to dark red. Each glass should look different; if not, add some more food coloring to the glasses, as appropriate. Line up the glasses on a table. You're ready to start!

Observe the glasses. Invite your child to observe the glasses. Discuss the use of color in their everyday surroundings. What color is their bedroom, for example? What are their favorite colors? Then ask your child about the relationship between color and mood. Older kids may be familiar with the use of color by advertisers and companies (who know that we often implicitly associate certain colors with certain emotions). For example, green is supposed to be calming (hospitals, waiting rooms).[19] Red is supposed to be fiery and energetic. Blue is associated with grief. Ask your child whether they can think of emotions associated with colors.

Taste and rank the samples. Now, ask your child to taste the liquid in the glasses, *telling them that some are sweeter than others.* Ask them to sip each one, and have them rate the sweetness. Record the results on a piece of paper.

Fooled you! Reveal the answer: the five cups were equally sweet. Chances are, your child will have rated the darker drinks as sweeter in taste. Once you have revealed that they were all of equal sweetness, discuss the reasons they were fooled. Ask them about processed foods they might eat, or have seen other people eating, that use color to enhance taste.

Game 15:
The Yogurt Game (Ages 6 and up)

Main message: This simple game makes the point that our sense of taste can be fooled by color (and particularly artificial coloring).

What you'll need:
Vanilla yogurt
Yellow (or orange) food coloring
Two small bowls

What to do:
Prepare the game. Without your child being able to see what you're doing, place an equal amount of vanilla yogurt in each bowl. To one bowl, add 1 or 2 drops of food coloring and mix well (the yogurt should have an appealing color and look distinctly different from the plain vanilla yogurt).

Taste test. Ask your child to taste the two bowls of yogurt and identify the flavors. Many kids will correctly identify the vanilla but incorrectly guess "apricot" or "orange" or "honey" for the other bowl.

Fooled you! After you've revealed the truth, ask your child why they thought that the yogurt had a different flavor. Ask them about the use of artificial colors in foods. What impact could this have on our experience of tasting those foods? Next time you're grocery shopping, have your child look at the labels on some of their favorite brands to see whether artificial colors have been used. They might be surprised: these additives are found in many common brands.

Older children may be interested in the difference between artificial colors (the most common ones include Red #40 and Yellow #5 and #6) and natural colors (from sources like beet juice, turmeric, and beta-carotene). You can also talk to your child about the relationship between artificial color additives and health. Some additives are proven or potential carcinogens.[20] Some studies have also found a link between artificial colors and hyperactivity in children, leading the British Food Standards Agency to advise parents of children with ADHD to remove all sources of artificial color from their children's diets.[21] The EU passed a law in 2008 requiring products containing artificial food dyes to carry labels warning of the potential impact on children's behavior. The United States FDA launched its own inquiry in 2011, prompting some brands to go "natural" and replace artificial coloring in their potato chips with natural coloring from a mix of beet juice, carrots, and purple cabbage.[22]

Variation: A fun variation to this experiment uses different colors of soda. Buy two or three sodas of distinctly different colors—such as cherry or lemon—as well as some plain, unflavored soda water. Prepare the soda in three cups, but add some orange food coloring to the plain soda. Then ask your child to taste it. Many kids will say that the orange drink (which is flavorless) tastes "orange"!

Top Tips for Eating Real Food (Not Kids' Food)

- **Do a family food inventory.** This will help identify which "kids' food" items you'd like to wean your child from. Take the inventory list when you go shopping!
- **Use gradual substitution to replace kids' food with "real foods."** Rather than going cold turkey, this gentler method works well, particularly with older kids.
- **Pick a long-term "healthy food" goal.** Make it modest (one that you'll stick to!).
- **Use the "rotation" rule.** Maximize the variety of the foods your child already likes.
- **Use the "try something new every day" rule.** Increase the variety in your child's diet. For more cautious eaters, try something new once per week.
- **Introduce your child to new foods** *before* **you serve them.** Kids can help pick, clean, and cook foods. Younger ones can simply look at the raw version before you work your kitchen magic!
- **Use seasonal foods as another variety booster.** This is an easy, fun way to make sure that you get maximum variety throughout the year.

Secret 6

Participation Works Better than Pressure

How well would your son play football if he learned about it by sitting in a classroom and watching a teacher talk about matches? Would your daughter learn to drive safely if she only watched videos telling her how important it was to "be safe"? Information is necessary, but certainly not enough! Our kids need to get out and practice until they have physically and mentally internalized the necessary skills.

The same is true with eating. Kids need to practice eating just as they would practice a sport (with you playing the role of coach). The more they follow their own interests and feel as if they are in control of their learning ("child-led," in parenting parlance), the more enthusiastic they are likely to be. Letting kids participate and take charge allows them to develop a sense of autonomy, mastery, and enjoyment that is key to life-long healthy eating.

This chapter explains some simple, fun activities you can use to foster child-led learning about healthy eating. My test families experimented with these techniques with lots of success. The activities range from gardening to meal planning, among other things, but share one goal: they encourage a child's involvement in eating rather than controlling what the child is eating. This is based on the simple premise that kids are generally more eager to eat foods if they've been involved in their preparation, whether through picking, buying, preparing, cooking, or meal planning.

Too much parental control usually backfires at some point. In fact, it can have long-term negative consequences: parents who overtly control their children's eating behaviors (by preventing them from eating certain foods or saying things like "Stop eating, you've had enough now" or "Keep eating, you haven't had enough") are more likely to foster disordered eating patterns, like dieting or binging.[1] Study after study proves that kids often show their independence by doing exactly the opposite of what we tell them to do. My favorite: in one experiment, parents were coached to prevent their children from eating an appealing-looking red snack food before leaving the room—after which most kids jumped on the candy and ate more of it than children whose parents had remained neutral.[2]

Offer age-appropriate choices

One simple strategy is to allow children to make age-appropriate choices. For example, ask your toddler which vegetable side dish they'd like with dinner: carrots or green beans? Or ask your child what size serving they would like. Kids who are allowed to determine how much they eat develop the sense of their own hunger and fullness cues, so they can start eating when hungry and stop eating when full. Serve small portions and allow them to ask for seconds.

Children will appreciate having their feelings about new foods acknowledged. Although you may feel that you are offering encouragement, they may see your multiple attempts at "forcing" them to eat new foods as pressure. This is a delicate balance. Remember that although parents decide what, when, and how food is served, children decide *whether* and *how much* to eat—but they should only make that decision after tasting everything that is served.

Asking older children to craft menus is a great way to make them feel like their food preferences matter. French schools do this on a regular basis; the child whose menu is selected as the "featured" menu for the entire school feels seriously proud! You can easily do this at home.

Another strategy is to ask children to talk about eating behaviors (rather than nutrition) or marketing, to let them in on the reasons behind your family eating routines. Allowing children to buy the food (for example, selecting "their" vegetables to take home) and involving older children in preparing dishes (which adults should then enjoy with gusto!) often also works wonders, as Roberta and Stacy, two moms in my test families, discovered:

Getting my three boys (ages 3, 5, and 7) involved in food shopping and prep is a big help. My kids love going to the grocery store and helping me pick out the fruits and vegetables. Often, I let them pick out a "funny fruit" to bring home and try. This is a really fun and exciting part of our shopping trip and a real treat for them. I let them search for a fruit or vegetable that we've never tried before (or rarely eat) that looks really funny or strange to them. They take pride in finding the oddest-looking one. Usually it ends up being an exotic tropical fruit (such as dragonfruit or prickly pear) and often they end up liking them. Sometimes they don't, but it doesn't matter all that much to them—it's the surprise of the experience that they really enjoy. Because they're the ones who choose the fruit, the experience is driven by them. This makes them eager to try it (never once have they turned down a taste of their "funny fruit," no matter how strange it looked on the inside). This has helped immensely in opening their minds and getting them to try new things.

—Roberta

Getting kids involved in the process is key. Last night I did a make-your-own salad. I put a big bowl of greens on the table along with small bowls of fruit (blueberries, mango, sliced green grapes, and dried cranberries), homemade croutons in star shapes, and salad dressing. (I purposely used fruit instead of veggies thinking it would be less daunting to them; I also did the shaped croutons to make it fun.) Only one of my kids will eat salad normally. But last night, they came running up to the table and started serving themselves. Even my 7-year-old, who doesn't like blueberries and mangoes, started piling them onto his salad. I was blown away! Why didn't I think of this sooner?! But I am not complaining. The fact that they were willing to eat salad, and ate it so enthusiastically, thrilled me to death. My 4-year-old twins even asked to have it again tonight for dinner. But my husband was cooking and didn't want to do make-your-own salad. Instead, he just put salad on their plates: mixed greens with salad dressing, no fruit. My 7-year-old didn't touch it. The twins nibbled at a few leaves. But overall, I'd say this standard salad was a no-go.

—Stacy

Of course, cooking itself can be a fun game for kids. Who doesn't like stirring the batter or squeezing juice out of fruit? You can try this at home or, if you're really lucky, find an organization that might be willing to provide cooking lessons at your school.

Get cooking!

Can you imagine a fourth-grade classroom full of kids happily eating kale and chard soup? Hard to imagine, isn't it? But it's a reality in the classrooms that Project CHEF (Cooking Healthy Edible Food) visits in my hometown, Vancouver. The brainchild of Barb Finley (a chef and former teacher), Project CHEF works with schools to provide hands-on education to primary school children. I recently had the pleasure of visiting a local classroom where Chef Barb was running one of her food education programs. What a treat! Barb and her team had transformed the classroom into an in-house cooking school, complete with a full-size cartoon mascot (a French chef!).

When I arrived, kids were sitting at tables, each with its own cooking zone (a hot plate), prep area (including knives, graters, and other useful utensils), and a vegetable tray full of the raw ingredients that the students—each divided into teams of five kids plus a volunteer parent helper—were going to transform into a delicious meal.

Minestrone was featured on the menu the day I visited—but not just any minestrone. This soup featured fresh kale from the school garden, local herbs, and an amazing collection of vegetables from farmers' markets, including Swiss chard. *How is this going to go over?* I wondered.

Barb started the class with a discussion of the recipe ingredients, asking students a series of questions that had them raising their hands eagerly. "How many vegetables are in this soup?" had everyone counting intently. The answers (ranging from 8 to 17) had everyone laughing, as Barb gently reminded kids how we define "vegetable": an edible plant (or part of an edible plant) without seeds—usually, the stem, root, or leaf of a plant. (This explains why tomatoes and avocadoes are technically fruits!)

The kids were even more attentive when Barb began making the soup, chopping the onion and then the other ingredients at her demo table, including some monstrous-looking carrots that had the kids gasping and laughing in appreciation.

"What's this one doing? The tango?" Barb asked, waving a gnarly, three-headed carrot at the class, followed by "We like vegetables with character, like this one. They have more flavor!" While Barb proceeded to chop and sample the "tango carrot" ("A good cook tastes her veggies!"), the class was utterly attentive: you could have heard a pin drop. When she slid the chopped onions into the olive oil, which sizzled away, the class reaction took even me by surprise.

"That's *so* cool!" shouted one boy.

"It smells *so* good!" said a girl at my table.

As Barb worked her way through the recipe, they—guided by the kids—learned about everything from "measurement versus estimation" to the secret of cooking onions successfully. You could sense they were eager to act on Barb's tips.

"How do I cut this sage up?" she asked. "With my hands—a cook's best instrument!" Handing the sage to a couple of children, she encouraged them: "Now smell your hands!" Thirty pairs of hands reached for the sage leaves on each table, and I noticed the parent volunteers doing the same.

As the delicious smell of Barb's simmering demonstration soup filled the room, the table teams started to make their own soups. This went much more smoothly than I expected, as each child had an assigned role (which changed every day throughout the week-long cooking class): Chopping, Supply, Washer, Drier, and Station "Meisters." Just like a line chef in a restaurant, each child had their responsibilities—a great way to avoid fights over who does what and encourage cooperation.

I admit that the chopping part of the class had me a bit worried. Thirty 8-year-olds wielding sharp knives? But I was reassured, as they had been trained by Barb and her team in "The Claw": a safe knife-handling technique. Sure enough, the kids folded their fingers back and hid their thumbs in a "claw" that safely held the veggies, while chopping everything from onions to garlic, carrots to tomatoes. Impressive!

Soon, seven soups were simmering away while the kids sat down to fill out worksheets. Barb took a few minutes to explain to me some of the secrets of success of her cooking program. First, kids make a commitment on the first day: *"Open mind, open mouth!"* They promise to try everything, and the week's menu is designed to have them tasting new things every day.

Barb explained that positive peer pressure and the thrill of preparing foods themselves really help in encouraging them to try new foods. She showed me the various lesson plans she had developed—all fully integrated with our educational curriculum. Interest has been so strong that Barb's classes now run five days a week, nine months of the year. In some schools, her team will set up for a month, training the entire primary school in age-appropriate cooking skills. When Project CHEF leaves the school, teachers have new ideas about ways to incorporate food and cooking into subjects ranging from English and science to art and geography.

While Barb and I chatted, the children washed, dried, and stored their cooking implements (ready for use by the next class) and then sat down to work on their learning logs, connecting the new learning to their lives. When they were finished, they began setting the tables with real china bowls and cutlery. Time to serve the soup! As it was lunchtime, everyone was feeling a little hungry. Meanwhile, curious faces peeked in the door (kids from other classes heading outside to play for lunchtime recess). You could tell by the looks on their faces that they would have liked to join us.

I sat down at a table with my own bowl and watched the kids around me. Many kids, Barb explained, didn't sit down and eat with their families. Surveys suggest that 70 percent of North American families don't eat together on a regular basis. Kids eat at the computer, in front of the TV, or in their bedroom. Eating together, she emphasized, was one of the best ways to ensure kids accepted—and liked—healthy food. That seemed to be the case at my table. Three of the kids polished off their bowls and asked for more. Even the more hesitant eaters ate at least half their bowls. No one refused it outright. Looking around the room, this seemed to be pretty representative. Success!

While they were eating, the kids talked about their "table talk topic" (officially "autumn vegetables," although we did drift off pretty quickly into talking about video games—but at least everyone was chatting happily!). Barb then stood to show the kids a pack of instant soup and read out the ingredients ("Artificial color! What do they do? Put a crayon in there?"), before asking kids why making soup at home was a good thing to do. The kids had lots of great answers: It tastes better! It costs less! It's healthier! It's more fun! I can put what I like in it! It was clear that some positive lessons had been learned.

Clean-up was fast: the kids filed up and scraped leftovers into the compost bucket (which they would later take out to the school compost heap, next to the garden). Bowls were neatly piled, cutlery dunked in the soapy water in big buckets, and everyone headed out to play.

Like many local food education organizations, Project CHEF exists because of the devotion of a small team of dedicated people. But as Barb's team showed, it only takes a few to make a huge difference.

If you do try cooking with your child at home, here are a few helpful tips:

- **Pick the right time.** Ideally, choose a time when everyone is well rested and not too hungry.
- **Pick an appropriate dish.** For young kids, pick something simple. For kids new to cooking, start with something familiar so they identify cooking with something they already enjoy.
- **Don't worry about the mess.** In fact, kids are great at cleaning up—ask them to help! Toddlers especially love wiping, sweeping, and cleaning counters and floors.
- **Find "sous chefs."** Invite a friend or relative over or keep your babysitter for an extra hour. It'll be less stress for everyone (especially you) if there is someone else to help oversee and clean up.
- **Stay upbeat.** Praise your child for tasks they do well. If the recipe goes awry, just laugh it off. Remind them that we eat several times a day, and each time is an opportunity to start over and learn something new. Your child will learn a good lesson: you can learn from your mistakes, and "there's no use crying over spilled milk"—especially in the kitchen.
- **Keep it simple.** Older kids may want to chop and stir but sometimes just a little bit of participation goes a long way. For example, my younger daughter loves tossing the salad with vinaigrette right before dinner. This gets her involved in food prep and has definitely encouraged her to eat salad.

Put a reluctant eater in charge

Project CHEF's classroom magic shows how powerful the simple act of cooking can be. Food is a sensual experience, and kids (even more than adults) are sensitive to physical impressions and sensations. Onions sizzling in a pan evoke an excited response from most kids—even those who might normally be indifferent or annoyed if an onion showed up in their soup. The simple act of handling vegetables helps "tame" them, making them less scary for kids. And kids are proud of what they create! Basically, children are much more willing to try a dish that they have a hand in creating—whether they're involved in choosing, smelling, touching, cutting, or cooking. (Babies, of course, can also play at cooking, even if it is limited to banging pots and pans with a wooden spoon to keep them busy.)

French families use this well-known fact to help kids conquer food dislikes. I've had many a proud French grandmother tell me about the personal food challenge she's orchestrated for her grandchildren. One was the mother of our friend Remi in France, who explained her savvy strategy upon being told by her 9-year-old grandson that he didn't like zucchini. Her response? They went and bought several pounds of zucchini at the local market, and then she helped him plan a zucchini-based menu for a family meal (which included sliced zucchini salad as a veggie starter, zucchini quiche, and zucchini cake for dessert!). The entire family enjoyed them and, despite his reluctance, her grandson admitted, "Maybe they aren't so bad after all."

One of my test families had a similarly inspiring experience. Lori's two daughters once held a long-standing aversion to "salad," a word they used to describe all green leafy vegetables. Lori, however, was determined to overcome their aversion to lettuce. She started by asking them to help prepare spinach salad one night, removing the stems and tearing the spinach leaves into bite-size pieces. To her surprise, they tore the leaves into much smaller pieces than Lori had been used to. Eureka! Lori also discovered that the kids didn't like salad with too much dressing.

She began serving the dressing separately, and even asked the kids to help make homemade dressings with flavors they liked. This grew into a full-blown "make-your-own salad" exercise. Her family ended up creating their own "Kids' Salad" recipe (with mandarin oranges, toasted almonds, and even sliced radishes). I've adapted this idea for one of the games at the end of this chapter. *Merci,* Lori!

Get out your green thumb

Another tactic you should try, if at all possible, is gardening (or the "green thumb gourmet program," as I call it). Gardening (whether at school or at home) helps kids in many ways: not only do they learn to recognize more fruits and vegetables, they're less likely to believe that vegetables taste bad—and so eat more veggies *and* a greater variety of veggies.[3]

Researchers believe this is because kids are more familiar with the vegetables; repeated exposure reassures them and piques their curiosity. Note: gardening can be as simple as growing cherry tomatoes and lettuce in little pots on your windowsill so the kids can create their own salad. The research on the "green thumb" effect is so amazing that I've included more information on gardening on my website (GettingToYum.com).

Finding the balance: How much should kids decide?

The other night we sat down to dinner with our daughters, who ate tomato-kale soup followed by roast fish and potatoes with one of our favorite carrot recipes, Vicious Carrots (page 225). We chatted and told stories about our day, and spent about 30 minutes at the table. My husband and I didn't have to spend any time acting as mealtime police and tempers never flared. My daughters (particularly Claire, who'd just turned 5) only required a couple of reminders to eat with their mouths closed and use their cutlery properly.

This sounds totally ordinary, right? When family mealtimes are working well, this *should* be totally ordinary—but all too often it's not. It certainly never used to be in our family. A few years ago (when our older daughter, Sophie, was 5), our mealtimes were often interrupted by tantrums about "yucky food," constant requests for pasta and buttered toast, food refusals, and even walking away from the table. Mealtime was one of the most dreaded moments in the day. My husband and I left the table feeling drained. The more we applied pressure— to sit at the table, to eat the foods that we offered, to use good table manners—the more our children resisted. We had created a bit of a battleground and weren't sure how to change the situation.

The secret to changing the situation seems counter-intuitive: less pressure, less fuss. No coercion, and certainly no force. Relax. I know this seems like frustrating advice when your kids are jumping up from the table or putting napkins on their heads or calling each other names or gag-choking on the food that you insist they taste or when you're following them around the house cajoling them for "one more bite." But believe me, there is another way.

Think of your parental role here as one of a coach. Observe and advise and help your child to learn eating skills. Don't take their food choices personally. Try to minimize or even avoid creating food fights; that way, food never becomes a power struggle but rather part of a routine, like brushing your teeth. Be nonchalant but cheerful about it. No coaxing, no hovering, no special routines or meals. Above all, if your child refuses to eat, take the food away without too much comment, but do not replace it with a requested favorite, no matter how hard that feels. They'll be hungrier at the next meal, which will work to your advantage.

Elizabeth Satter, one of America's best-known kids' food writers, terms this approach the "division of responsibility": parents are responsible for when kids eat and what is served; kids choose how much and whether they eat any particular item. The only thing I would add to Satter's approach is the idea that kids have to *taste* everything that is served, although they are not required to eat it. Of course, this approach begs the question of food likes and dislikes: how do we get children to actually *like* these foods? Repeated exposure (repeated practice) to vegetables is key, and this strategy is discussed in detail in Secret 2.

There's another key role for parents: helping your kids develop the internal self-motivation to *want* healthy food. Your children should learn to eat healthy food because they *want* to, not because you *make* them. But the key to success is doing this in a low-pressure environment, which is the focus of the next chapter. Before that, here are some more fun games to foster your child's participation in building healthy eating habits.

Fun games for getting your child involved

For many kids, games won't be necessary: they'll be having enough fun helping you cook and bake. But the games listed below add an extra twist that will keep things interesting. And some of the games will be useful for reluctant kids. Game 16: The Mixing Game, for example, is designed to help kids who don't like eating combinations of foods of different textures.

Game 16:
The Mixing Game (Ages 2 and up)

Main message: What should you do if a child doesn't want to mix foods or let them touch on a plate? Put the child in charge. Even better: call it a game! This game will teach your child to enjoy different textures by allowing them to take charge of mixing food for themselves. It develops their "mixing" skills so they'll eat foods with combined textures more easily.

Note: The following steps should be carried out on consecutive days. If more than a week has gone by, you might want to go back a step.

Day 1: Mixing fun. Start with a simple mixing game that doesn't necessarily involve food you're going to eat. Provide your child with at least two bowls, each containing a separate ingredient. Some simple ideas for ingredients to use include: two varieties of rice (brown rice and white rice); two colors of rice (you can use diluted food coloring on dry white rice—just be sure to let it dry!); or two distinct types of dried beans (kidney beans and chickpeas). (Note: beware of a choking hazard with all types of dried beans.) Give your child a third bowl for mixing, a utensil for dipping and transferring, and a spoon for stirring. Then let your child mix away! As they do so, encourage them to notice how the mixing creates nice colors and interesting swirl effects. Encourage your child to touch the mixed ingredients with their hands. Ask them how it feels.

Day 2: Mixing a favorite dish. Prepare the ingredients for a dish your child normally likes. Show your child how you combine the ingredients to make the dish. If possible, have your child add the ingredients together and do the stirring. When it comes time to serve, remember to announce that this was a dish your child helped to mix. You may even want to ask if your child would like to help with serving.

Day 3: Mixing at snack-time. Gradually introduce mixing at snack-time. Set the table with separate bowls of items your child normally likes. An easy option is plain yogurt with strawberry jam (or another flavor they like). Place one spoon in each bowl and then provide your child with a third, empty bowl and another spoon. Ask your child to taste each ingredient separately, and then encourage them to mix up their own fruit yogurt to enjoy as a snack.

Day 4: A new twist on an old favorite. Prepare a dish that your child usually likes to eat. Choose one added ingredient that changes the dish somewhat, but not too much (such as adding ¼ teaspoon ground cinnamon to applesauce or 1 teaspoon parsley to pasta and cheese). Ask your toddler to combine the ingredients themselves, stirring and serving as before.

Day 5: The "Make It Yourself Mixed-Up Meal." Now that your child has some confidence in their new mixing skills, why not have a "mixed-up meal"? Choose a dish that's easy for a child to put together. For example, serve pitta bread and place bowls on the table with ingredients your child likes to eat (whatever that might be—if it's blueberries and cream cheese, so be it!). Allow them to stuff their own pitta. They'll be much more likely to eat it if they're allowed to do it themselves.

Game 17:
Make-Your-Own Kids' Salad Game (Ages 4 and up)

Main message: Kids can learn to love salad if they're allowed to take control. Warning: this can result in some very strange salads!

What you'll need:
1 small head of lettuce
3 of your child's favorite fresh fruits or veggies

What to do: Explain to your child that they're going to get to create their own personalized kids' salad, just for them. Ask them to name three favorite fruits and vegetables. Next time you're shopping, bring your child along and ask them to pick out their choices. Once home, have your child help prepare the items (younger children can wash, older children can peel and chop). Have your child wash a few leaves of lettuce and tear the leaves into bite-size pieces to make the base of the salad. Then have your child layer their choice of fruits and vegetables on top. You'll get some weird and wonderful creations, but at least you'll be able to say your child likes salad!

Optional: Dressing is their choice, too. You might want to try my homemade Classic Vinaigrette (page 365).

Top Tips For Letting Your Kids Lead

- **Offer age-appropriate choices.** Giving kids completely free rein in the kitchen isn't usually a great idea, but allowing specific choices ("Would you like dried cranberries or blueberries as a fun topping for your salad?") gets kids motivated.
- **Get cooking.** Get your kids involved stirring, mixing, pouring, etc.—this works for kids of all ages. Older kids in particular will be more eager to eat the dishes they have prepared themselves.
- **Put reluctant eaters in charge.** If your child has a dislike for a particular food, they might benefit from a cooking challenge: ask them to find a recipe that makes the food appetizing and serve it to the family.
- **Decide on your family's "division of responsibility."** Parents decide when the family eats and what is served; kids decide whether to eat and how much. This works well for younger kids, but as kids get older, involving the kids more makes sense (older children may enjoy meal planning one day a week, for example).
- **Try gardening.** Growing, cultivating, and picking fruits and vegetables have a wonderful effect on many picky eaters. If you don't have a garden, try visiting one or starting one at your kids' school or in the community. Farmers' markets are also great places to introduce kids to vegetables.

Secret 7

Mindful Eating Is Mealtime Magic

The "Ig Nobel" Prize (a spoof sponsored by the scientific humor magazine *Society for the Annals of Improbable Research*) is one of the most iconic—and ironic—prizes awarded to scientists. Brian Wansink, professor of marketing research at Cornell University and former prizewinner, certainly has produced research that, as the Society says, "makes people laugh and then think."

The experiment that won Wansink the prize was deceptively simple.[1] He asked his (adult) research subjects to come into a classroom set up as a restaurant and enjoy a bowl of tomato soup. The participants—four to a table—chatted away, ate their soup, and then left the room when they were done eating. That, they thought, was that.

Except it wasn't that straightforward. Wansink called them back later to inform them how much they had eaten and to reveal the trick he'd used at the table: what participants didn't know was that two of the four bowls were attached to a tube beneath the table that slowly (very slowly) refilled the bowls. The people eating from these "bottomless bowls" ate 73 percent more soup than those eating from normal bowls, yet they didn't rate themselves as any fuller than those eating from normal bowls.

"This research shows that we eat with our eyes and not with our stomach," said Wansink. "The cues around us have a huge influence on not only what we eat, but also how much we eat and when we feel full."[2]

Wansink, who has studied our eating behaviors for decades, has had much experience at proving to disbelieving audiences that overeating is often unconscious. As explored in his book *Mindless Eating: Why We Eat More Than We Think*, we are prompted to overeat by everything from the size of packaging, plates, and containers to the names and labels of foods, lighting and colors, shapes and smells, and the organization of our cupboards. Kids serve themselves 74 percent more soda when using short, wide glasses, and people eat more ice cream when using bigger bowls.[3]

But Wansink's work also shows us how we can turn this around: by being mindful of the choices we make. Simple strategies—such as using smaller plates and bowls, or reorganizing cupboards to hide junk foods at the back—can have impressive results for people trying to lose weight. Simply put: making poor-quality food choices more inconvenient is a great way to help people be healthier.[4]

Certain trigger foods—simply by their presence in the cafeteria line or on the table—can encourage kids to consume more healthy fruits and veggies.[5] In one experiment done by British researchers (which echoes our familiar flavor approach from Secret 1: Kids Can *Learn* to Love Healthy Foods), placing a familiar fruit (like a banana) on the table next to a novel fruit (a guava) meant children were more likely to try the new food.[6] Changing the environment is also an important tactic (well understood by marketers and food companies).[7] Mood lighting, bigger plates, supersize containers, attractive names—all encourage us to eat more. We can turn these tactics on their head, says Wansink, and make healthy eating "mindless" by developing daily routines and environments that promote eating the right amounts of healthy foods without thinking (or obsessing) about it. For example, serve new foods in very small containers (or even on a spoon) to make them less overwhelming in appearance for children. A simple placemat or tablecloth often works wonders, setting the stage for settling in at the table rather than eating on the run.

Many of these tactics are intended to "automate" healthy eating behaviors, just as Wansink suggests. As my test families found out (and as research verifies), these are useful tactics for improving your families' eating habits. But there's more to healthy eating than that.

From mindless to mindful eating

The phrase "mindful eating" might sound a little new agey, but bear with me for a moment. The slow and thoughtful eating championed by mindful eating advocates isn't really a Western rediscovery of Eastern philosophies. It's the rediscovery of something that our great-grandparents used to know—and that some (like the French) haven't yet forgotten.

Food is deeply sensual. When we eat a piece of food, our enjoyment is affected by our senses of smell, touch, sight, taste, and even hearing. Don't believe me? Try eating a piece of your favorite cake with your nose plugged or with earplugs in. Or try taking a bite and swallowing quickly, without chewing. You'll discover that eating slowly, using all of our senses, is the key to finding pleasure in food. In fact, the French have built their entire national school food curriculum around this insight: that engaging food with all of your senses makes you a more thoughtful—and thus better—eater. You'll be better attuned to your own sense of fullness (satiety). You'll appreciate the subtle tastes of foods more (and not need the flavor hit of overly salty, sugary, fatty foods).

But eating is not purely physical, and it's not only about nutrition. It's also social and, thus, emotional. Pleasurable taste is important, but sharing food (or eating alone) also affects us emotionally. The difference between the preferred comfort foods of North American men (steak, pasta, burgers) and women (cookies, chocolate, and ice cream) is about *emotional* connections to food. As Brian Wansink observes, "Men prefer meal-related comfort foods because they make them feel special and well taken care of. Women, on the other hand, *don't* think of these as comfort foods. These foods reminded them of work—cooking and clean-up. Women much preferred the convenience of snack foods. Eating ice cream from the container equals no cooking and no clean up."[8]

How do we create positive associations with healthy food? The family meal is one of the best tools we have. All around the world, people celebrate formal gatherings—celebrations and festivities, christenings and funerals—by coming together to share meals. We do this because meals have the power to make us feel good—emotionally as well as physically. You know the wonderful, relaxed feeling you have after a celebratory family meal? Imagine if you felt that way every day! Not because of overeating, but because the busy world stopped for just a few minutes and you simply sat and enjoyed your food and the pleasure of being together with your family. This would have sounded unrealistic before I spent time in a country where family food culture is a priority: family meals, for the French, are akin to what Buddhists term a "practice." For the French, having a good meal is like going for a good run or getting a massage or doing a great yoga session. They feel relaxed, both emotionally and physically satisfied. The French even try to cultivate this in their children. Here is a quote from the Town Hall of Versailles (outside of Paris) that describes their philosophy about school lunches:

> Mealtime is a particularly important moment in a child's day. Our responsibility is to provide children with healthy, balanced meals; to develop their sense of taste; to help children, complementing what they learn at home, to make good food choices without being influenced by trends, media, and marketing; and to teach them the relationship between eating habits and health. But above all else, we aim to enable children to spend joyful, convivial moments together, to learn savoir-vivre ["the art of living"], to make time for communication, social exchange, and learning about society's rules—so that they can socialize and cultivate friendships.

Food is (a little bit like) Family therapy

Families need to socialize and cultivate friendships. Families need to spend joyful moments together, and to make time for communication and conversation. Eating is, in other words, a little bit like family therapy. Why does all of the research show that kids do better in a family that eats meals together, with positive rituals and routines? It's because eating is a way for families to negotiate togetherness, to reaffirm relationships. This is not always straightforward. It's about finding the right balance between love and limits. It's about doing your best and letting go of guilt when sometimes (inevitably) you make mistakes. It's about parents searching for their own personal "Zen of family eating": both an acceptance of where your kids are at and supportive, yet non-judgmental persistence with your teaching. It's about sensing when less is more: less pressure, less fuss, less rush, less choice, and (sometimes) less praise. It's about being detached enough to act, rather than react. Most important, it's about love. Feeding is parenting: kids must have their emotional needs met (and have the right balance struck between "love and limits") to do a good job with eating.

> *Over years of cooking, I've begun to understand one basic principle: it's about "the love." My daughter always brings up the love in a recipe. She will look at a dish of sweet potato polenta with poached shrimp and demand, matter-of-factly, "Hey, Dad, did you remember the love?" In our house, "the love" isn't just some kind of sentimental way of saying we care about what we feed our kids. It is making sure the food is something they're going to want to eat. It's the skill of a chef who knows how to sell what he makes—how to market it, present it, and make it shine.*
> —*Jason Hammel*[9]

Jason (a trained chef) intuitively knows what researchers have proven: if food is prepared with love and served in a warm, loving environment, children are much more likely to eat it. This is particularly the case when it comes to learning to eat new foods.[10] If you find sources of pleasure and joy for kids in healthy food, it will become *their* comfort food.

I'm not saying that love will immediately solve all of your kid's eating problems! And I'm certainly not accusing you of not providing enough love at the table. It's simply a reminder: in addition to education and exposure to healthy foods, the most important ingredient of all is gentle encouragement. This is hard to remember when standing over a toddler with pursed lips at dinnertime, I know. But do try to remember to show the love you feel, particularly at those tough moments.

By mentioning love, I also don't mean that you should avoid conflict altogether (which leads some parents to short-order cook and let their kids eat whatever they want). Creating a healthy family food culture sometimes requires a bit of tough love to get to the point where you can be joyful at the table together. Industrial food culture presents families with new challenges that are very different from those previous generations have faced: an over-abundance of high-calorie, low-nutrition foods, with no innate controls about how to respond in moderation (and in fact many pressures to do just the opposite).[11] This is not just an issue in the wealthiest countries. Countries as far-flung as Brazil, Mexico, India, and China have similar problems. The good news: there's something you can do about it!

Of course, it probably won't be a quick fix. Creating a healthy family food culture takes time, requiring you to establish—and stick to—core values that may run counter to fast food culture.[12] Doing so might give you some short-term pain, but the long-term gain will be worth it. You'll be giving your children the gift of the values and self-motivation to eat well—for life—by teaching them to be competent, autonomous eaters (without bribes, rewards, nagging, or any other external incentives). These values will vary between families. For some, eating well is about personal health. For others, it might be about the environment. For others, it may be about spirituality, about treating the body as a temple or following time-honored religious precepts.[13] Finding and sharing these core values with your children as they grow will be one of the best ways in which your family food culture becomes an enduring source of joy.

Tell Funny jokes

You've probably heard (too many times) how family meals are the best preventive medicine for our kids. Children who eat with their families on a regular basis are less likely to be overweight or suffer from depression, and are more likely to do well in school. The challenge for many of us—including my family—is that life is simply really, really busy. If you have two working parents (our case) with no help at home (also our case), mealtimes are often a seriously stressful scramble at the end of the day.

To be frank, family mealtimes aren't always that much fun even if people have the time. Between siblings nit-picking at one another, complaints about what happened at school, stressed-out parents, and the all-too-usual comments on the food ("I don't like this!"), they can actually be a real downer.

So how can you put fun back into the family food equation? At our house, we've found that a little fun goes a long way. Of course, "fun" will mean different things to different people. Different approaches will work for kids of different ages. For some people, this may mean telling jokes (my test families had a lot of fun telling carrot jokes during the week they were testing carrot recipes). Other people might want to play simple games. Your goal is to create a light-hearted atmosphere of trust, acceptance, and engagement. I don't have to tell you that kids love jokes, especially ones that they can master and tell themselves. If family mealtimes have been tense, you can defuse them almost immediately by telling a joke—even if it's as silly as these.

The jokes don't have to be brilliant. In fact, they can often be a little time-worn. They range from the obvious . . .

Q: What game do elephants love to play?
A: Squash.

to the subtle ...

    Q: Why did the carrot win a prize?
    A: Because he was out standing in his field.

or even the risqué ...

    Q: Why did the tomato blush?
    A: Because he saw the salad dressing.

Why slow = success

What are the advantages of eating slowly? It allows more time for kids to describe their reactions to food (one of the most important elements in taste training). Rather than "yuck" or "I don't like that," encourage your child to describe their sensations: "sour" or "slippery" or "rough." By talking about how food feels, kids learn to get over their first reactions to food, which are often feelings of caution or suspicion.

Eating slowly has another advantage: it allows the "fullness" signals produced by your stomach time to reach your brain (this takes somewhere around 20 minutes). It's a natural way to avoid overeating.[14] Another great way to avoid overeating is to ask your children to gauge their fullness. Japanese tradition holds that it is best to stop eating when you are 80 percent full. French parents ask their children "Are you still hungry?" rather than "Are you full?"—a subtle but important distinction.[15] It's an important lesson to teach your child, one that will help them naturally resist overly large portion sizes, which have increased hugely in recent years. (In the mid-1970s, the average sugary beverage was about 13 ounces; today, it's closer to 20 ounces. Yikes![16])

How many kids eat a hurried dinner in the car on the way to after-school activities, or gobble lunch at school before running outside to play? By doing this, our children are learning that food is fuel, that it doesn't matter what you eat as long as you fill up, that eating is an interruption in the day and a distraction from the productive, interesting, fun things in life. What a lesson! Consider weaning yourself off the "food is fuel" approach by committing to at least one slow family meal per week, even if it's a lazy weekend breakfast.

Changing your family eating habits will happen slowly, so you might as well enjoy the journey. Remember that although each change is incremental, they really add up. Our family is a good example. My two daughters are now good eaters, but they weren't always that way. In particular, my elder daughter, Sophie, had a long list of "no go" foods when she was younger, including sandwiches, macaroni and cheese, and anything white and creamy (yes, even ice cream). Efforts to introduce these foods would be met with serious opposition, to put it mildly. Her younger sister, Claire, wasn't much better.

These days if you mention the word "Roquefort" to Claire she looks happy, as if someone had offered ice cream (and she *loves* ice cream). Taking a little morsel of cheese, she'll place it in her mouth and slowly savor it, clearly delighting in the salty, slightly tangy, creamy taste. The older and the moldier the cheese, the better. We once found weeks-old suspicious-looking leftover cheese in the fridge, glisteningly humid, with the delightful odor of long-forgotten wet socks. Undeterred, Claire delicately tested her serving and declared it "yummy," then requested seconds. I'm kind of amazed by this, but my French husband, in-laws and friends were supremely unimpressed. "She likes Roquefort? *Mais bien sur!*" they responded, with a shrug. "*C'est normal!*"

Most French kids love all kinds of dairy products; the French have, after all, invented more than 300 varieties of cheese. In fact, French kids even eat cheese every day at school lunch (rather than drink milk). In a nation of cheese lovers, one more Roquefort-loving kid is not going to get anyone's attention. When I try to explain to my French in-laws that I wouldn't eat anything except bright orange Cheddar cheese when growing up, and that knowingly selling moldy food (much less feeding it to children) could be considered a criminal offense where I come from, I get blank looks.

I now know that this is not miraculous. The reason my daughter loves Roquefort is simple: she was *taught* to love Roquefort. More precisely, she was given the skills to teach herself to love it. No one forced her. In fact, most parents know that force usually backfires. Even the youngest children can demonstrate a will of steel when confronted with a food they've decided will not pass their lips. Research suggests that forcing children to eat actually results in lower vegetable intakes, and a higher incidence of eating disorders later on in life. In experiments, kids who are *less* pressured will eat *more*, and kids who are forced to eat may develop dislikes for those foods that can endure into adulthood.[17]

Parents who are good role models are likely to have better success. Begin by asking yourself these questions: *Why* do you eat? What is the purpose of eating—for yourself, as well as for your children? Do you eat meals on the run? In the car? At the counter? How much is food a priority in your day? If food is a busy interruption, an after-thought, or a nuisance, your children will absorb that message.

Now consider this: what if you ate food slowly, savoring and talking about it, rather than rushing through the meal? What if meals (and, if you can swing it, a family meal) were one of the highlights of the day? What if preparing food together was something fun, a moment of connection, rather than a scramble at six o'clock, when you're fending off hungry kids from snacking while feeling stressed about the hassle of getting something on the table? What if trying new things was a shared family food adventure rather than a battle of wills?

All of this can be summed up in a simple formula:

Less pressure + less stress + more family
fun at the table = more success

This formula assumes that picky eating is partly a power struggle. Of course, some kids have underlying health issues. For most kids, though, resistance to healthy food is psychological, not physiological. It might seem counter-intuitive, but putting kids in charge of healthy eating, at an age-appropriate level, may defuse resistance and eliminate power struggles. That's the Zen of family eating—for kids of all ages.

Game 18:
The Slow Food Experiment (Ages 6 and up)

Main message: This game helps your child learn that the pace at which we eat our food influences how much we enjoy it. In general, the slower we eat, the better.

What you'll need: A soft food that your child likes, such as cheesecake.

What to do:
Taste test eating quickly. Pick a calm moment during the day (snack-time or dessert after dinner) when there is nowhere to rush off to. Give a teaspoon of your chosen food to your child and ask them to swallow it without chewing. Ask them how it felt.

Taste test eating slowly. Ask your child to take another spoonful, this time chewing slowly. Ask them to compare the difference in taste during chewing and after swallowing. Most children discover that chewing actually releases flavor. Remind your child of the relationship between smell and taste. Ask, "How might chewing release smells that affect how you taste things?"

Chat about it. Talk to your child about times when they eat quickly. Ask why eating slowly may be a good thing for other reasons (social or safety-related). Ask whether your family might need reminders to eat slowly at certain times and what form these reminders might take. Younger kids may even enjoy having a secret code word or signal to use! For older children, you might want to explore the concept of mindful eating, as discussed earlier in this chapter.

Game 19:
The Same Food Three Ways Experiment
(Ages 4 and up)

Main message: This is a wonderful experiment that one of the readers of *French Kids Eat Everything* designed to make variety fun for kids. (*Thanks, Stacy!*) It's a way to talk about food—where it comes from and all the different ways that it can be eaten. The idea is to provide one food in three different forms, to make variety fun and interesting for kids. In this example, spinach is used.

Note: the Slow Food movement uses this idea for their taste-testing classes, too, but asks kids to try three types of apple, or three types of chocolate, and describe the appearance, tastes, textures, and aromas. You don't have to do this with spinach—pick anything you like!

Stacy, the mom who designed this experiment, had this to say about her experience:

A few days ago, I decided to try this game with spinach—one of the foods that my 4-year-old twins, Jamie and Reese, claim to not like. This time, I prepared a green smoothie with a large handful of spinach, a sliced banana, a couple spoonfuls of vanilla yogurt, whole milk, and crushed ice. Next, I sliced pieces of baguette and spread it with spinach walnut pesto (something that they like on pasta but I've never tried serving on bread before). On each plate, I placed one fresh spinach leaf. I also added a second piece of baguette with real butter (I wanted to make sure that there was one item that they would be happy about).

When I called the twins to come to the table for our experiment, Jamie was the first to arrive. He looked at his plate and said, "Oh, yummy!" (Not kidding!) Reese, who was trailing behind, sat down without saying anything positive or negative. I took it as a good sign. Jamie started by picking up the spinach leaf and asking, "What's this? Salad?" I said, "It's spinach." Then I explained that we were doing a food-tasting experiment. He proceeded to pop the spinach leaf in his mouth. Reese followed his lead. Next came the smoothies. They didn't say much as they sipped but seemed happy. I then explained the gist of the lesson: I had served them spinach in three different ways— a plain leaf, puréed in pesto, and blended up in a drink. I said, "See how the smoothie is green? That's spinach!" Then I added, looking straight at Jamie, "You say you don't like spinach. But you do!" He said, "Yeah, you're right!" Finally, the baguette with the pesto. This was the one that I was most skeptical about. Even though they eat the pesto on pasta all the time, I wondered whether they would reject it this way. Nope—wrong again.

Every time that I've done "Food Three Ways," it's been a success. I think they like the "experiment" aspect of it, without any pressure to eat it. My kids don't always eat everything, but they almost always taste it without prodding.

—Stacy

What you'll need: Pick one of the fruits or vegetables from the recipe section in the second half of this book. Each fruit or vegetable has several recipe variations; pick two that you like. I recommend that you pick zucchini and make Melt-in-your-mouth Zucchini Purée (page 284) and Roasted Zucchini with Cumin (page 285), reserving some zucchini to serve in thin, raw slices.

What to do: Pick a time when your child is not too tired and not too hungry, but still likely to be interested in food; snack-time is a good bet for most kids. Tell the kids you'll be doing an experiment, and invite them to the table. Have the three different versions of the food ready and invite the kids to try them in any order they like. Use the taste-testing ideas from Secret 1: Kids Can *Learn* to Love Healthy Foods (page 33) to encourage them to describe and then taste the food. Ask them to pick a favorite; usually even the most dubious kids will be tempted by this idea. Reluctant eaters will be encouraged if you try everything yourself. Remember: treat any refusals with as much nonchalance as you can muster.

Game 20:
The Taste of Place Game (Ages 6 and Up)

Main message: This game introduces your child to the concept of *terroir*, a French word that roughly translates as "taste of place." Simply, *terroir* is the relationship between food culture, climate, and landscape: different places produce different types of foods. You can use examples from your region or well-known examples from elsewhere, such as maple syrup from Canada, and Parmesan from Italy.

What you'll need: 1 or more ripe vegetables or fruits, preferably local (easiest if you do this in the summertime, when local foods are ripe for harvesting).

What to do:
Introduce the concept of *terroir* using a simple explanation. Tell your child you're going to do a taste test of fruits or vegetables from nearby and far away.
Visit a market (optional). *If* you have a chance, take your child to a local farmers' market to have them pick fruits or vegetables to use in this exercise and to talk to the farmers. Then head to the

supermarket and buy the same fruits or vegetables from another region (chances are you may find one from another country). Good choices include tomatoes, peaches, plums, (podded) peas, beans, or peppers.

Taste test. Wash the two fruits or vegetables and peel or slice them as appropriate. Present them on separate plates (it's a good idea to use different-colored plates if you can so you can tell which is which). Ask your child to sample them, comparing their color, texture, smell, and taste.

Chat about it. Talk about why the two fruits or vegetables are different. Older kids might be interested to learn that nutrients are higher in local foods that haven't been transported long distances or stored for long amounts of time. This means more freshness and flavor, as well as more nutrients and a lower environmental impact. Try following up by cooking a recipe that features only local ingredients. This is a fun summer project for kids—particularly if you put them in charge!

Top Tips for Zen Family Eating

- **Slow down.** The more slowly we eat, the better food tastes. In general, slower eating encourages more moderate consumption: the more slowly we eat, the less likely we're to overeat.
- **Lighten up.** Make it a routine to tell funny jokes at the table; a happier mood makes for better eaters.
- **Aim for mindful rather than mindless eating.** Use the techniques described in this chapter to encourage kids to be aware of the foods they eat; this will improve their vocabulary as well as their eating skills!
- **Grow your own food or seek out people who do.** Growing your own food is calming, inspiring, and rewarding for the whole family. School and community gardens, or your own backyard, are great places

for the whole family. Plants in pots on the balcony (an herb garden, with tomatoes in the summer) are a fun, low-maintenance option.

- **Strike the right balance between love and limits.** Gentle, authoritative parenting at mealtimes will get the best results in the long run.

- **Treat mealtimes as family bonding time.** Kids are likelier to eat healthier meals if they have their emotional needs met. The family table is one of the best places to do this—in a low-pressure atmosphere.

Step-by-Step Strategies for Kids of All Ages

Babies: Feeding Maximum Variety with Minimum Fuss

It seems to be taken for granted in the United States that kids will innately dislike vegetables. But French mothers assume they will like them—and they do! I believe taste and appreciation of good and healthy foods, and curiosity for a wide variety of foods, can be learned and taught, and the earlier the better. Even my pediatrician was somewhat surprised that Pablo [18 months old] ate vegetables of all colors easily and thus didn't need to take a vitamin supplement.

—Hélène

When Hélène Garcia, a French-born mom living in Los Angeles, began feeding solid foods to her baby, Pablo, she did what comes naturally. She assumed he would be as interested in food as she was. Rather than treating it as a chore, she thought of feeding Pablo as a wonderful way for the two of them to bond and to simply have fun together.

She also knew one very important thing: the more you expose your baby to a range of flavors, textures, and tastes, the more likely your baby is to grow up enjoying a wide variety of healthy foods.[1] Simply put, if you feed them white rice cereal, they're more likely to grow up liking white bread. But if, as Hélène did, you feed them leeks and watercress (6 months), and then salmon and kale purée (12 months), you'll have a baby who loves eating salmon-wrapped leeks *au gratin* (18 months)—as Pablo did.

The French don't have a monopoly on this approach, of course. Parents in many other countries take a more adventurous approach to children's food than is found in countries like the US, Britain, or Canada. Mexican and Indian children eat spicy foods early on![2] Italian parents start their babies off with *Brodo* (page 364), a delicious vegetable stock.

These parents know that introducing maximum variety (adapted to your baby's personal preferences and eating type— more on this below) with minimum fuss helps your kids get off to a great start. Luckily, most babies are naturally curious and treat food as one more way to explore the world. I know that introducing variety might seem daunting, but remember that the eating habits your baby learns in their first few years will shape their eating habits throughout life—affecting mental and physical health.[3] What you teach your baby to eat will shape their preferences as a toddler, which in turn will affect what they are likely to eat as a preschooler, which shapes their palate as an adolescent and adult. Learning to like new foods isn't always a straightforward trajectory, but the effort you put in is—I promise—worth it.

Feeding your baby should be fun. It's a wonderful way to teach them about interacting with the world. Think of feeding your baby as a form of teaching—in which they're learning all sorts of fun new tastes, colors, and textures—the building blocks of their relationship with food. The more enthusiastic yet relaxed you are, the more smoothly this will happen.

Remember, by introducing lots of variety now, you're saving yourself time and stress later. The sooner your baby joins you at the table at mealtimes and starts eating baby versions (puréed, mashed, or chopped) of homemade, healthy adult food (without added salt and preservatives), the less work it will be for you. "One family, one meal" is a good motto to live by, and the recipes in this book will give you ideas of how you can take one vegetable and present it in age-appropriate ways for all members of your family.

When I launched an appeal for stories on my Facebook page, Catherine wrote to describe how she had approached food diversification for her two young sons. Working full-time with long workdays, she decided to cook during the weekends and freeze meals to be reheated during the week. When each boy was 6 months old, Catherine started cooking up purées with all of the vegetables she could find: green beans, cauliflower, carrots, zucchini, leeks, artichokes, broccoli, pumpkins, potatoes, sweet potatoes, even chicory! The purées contained a little potato and/or milk, so that the tastes of the veggies weren't too intense. Catherine did the same thing for fish purées so that her sons learned to like a wide range of fish early on. Her sons did go through the typical "no" phase at the age of 2, but Catherine held firm (not easy every day!), and the "no" phase ended— about 6 months after it started for one son and nearly a year later for her other son. By this time, Catherine happily wrote, they were "eating like adults." This doesn't mean that her children eat absolutely everything (yet)! Now 13, one son still dislikes yogurt; his 10-year-old brother dislikes cheese and butter. But that's okay: Catherine encourages them and tells them they will eventually learn to like it. Catherine summed up her philosophy:

> *The point is that none of us would spontaneously choose zucchini instead of a good chocolate cake. But we can learn not to always choose the cake, and we can also learn to appreciate zucchini. Except if we've been taught that we can always choose the chocolate cake.*
>
> *—Catherine*

Luckily, as Catherine found out, your baby is on your side. Most babies will try almost any flavor you give them when they're young. They're naturally curious: just as they go for the new toy in the room, they'll go for the new color on the plate. That doesn't mean they'll eat it! You may have to introduce it several times before they accept it. Remember: variation is normal. What and how much your baby will want to eat will vary from day to day. Your baby's food likes and dislikes will also vary. Children will have a new favorite food that they may like for a week or two and then refuse to touch. My younger daughter, Claire, loved oatmeal for several months, wouldn't touch it for a few months after that, and then started devouring it again. Keep re-offering the foods from time to time, and they'll rotate back into your child's preferences again. This may have the added benefit of increasing your child's interest in food, as you'll be appealing to their natural love of novelty.

Which first foods should I start with?

The million-dollar question for new parents is "What first foods should I give my baby?" Basically, science doesn't provide an answer. The most recent review by top American scientists simply notes that "There is no evidence for a benefit to introducing foods in any specific sequence or at any specific rate. However, it is generally recommended that first solid foods be single-ingredient foods and that they be started one at a time. The order of introduction of complementary foods is not critical. Combination foods may be given to older infants after tolerance for the individual components has been established."[4]

Translation? A mix of parental intuition and common sense is going to be your best guide. I'll explore some suggestions in this chapter, drawing on the French approach (as recommended by French pediatricians), because it emphasizes variety more than many other food cultures. Note that I don't agree with everything that the French do. For example, despite all of the research demonstrating the advantages of breast-feeding, France has some of the lowest breast-feeding rates in the industrialized world, and if French mothers do breast-feed, they typically stop at 2 months.

However, their approach to food diversification for babies is something that lots of parents around the world could learn from, and that's what I focus on here.

As you decide what to feed your baby, I'd also suggest drawing on your own cultural heritage combined with common sense (and discussions with your health-care provider as appropriate). Dr. Jatinder Bhatia (Chief Neonatologist at Georgia Health Science University and member of the American Academy of Pediatrics Committee on Nutrition) argues that Canadian and American guidelines contain a cultural bias that fails to reflect our ethnic diversity.[5] He recommends feeding mild curries to babies.

You might be happy to know that your baby has been learning about flavors since even before starting solid foods—and even before birth![6] Foods eaten by women during pregnancy flavor the amniotic fluid and thus influence babies' taste preferences.[7] If you eat lots of strong-flavored greens (such as rocket) during your pregnancy, chances are that your child will love these, too. (I realize now that my love of grilled cheese sandwiches—one of the only things I could eat during my first pregnancy without throwing up—was probably not the best tactic for raising a happy omnivore!)

What you eat also flavors your breast milk, so babies continue to encounter new flavors early on. Some studies have even found that varying the flavor of formula (for bottle-fed babies) can also increase the acceptance of specific foods later on.[8] What does this mean? Simply put, although we are born with certain preferences, our experiences are profoundly important in shaping what we like to eat.[9] The best time in a child's life to shape their food preferences is before the age of 2, when most children hit the "no" stage and many also develop temporary neophobia (fear of new foods). Knowing this, French parents (like many parents around the world) aim to develop their baby's love of a wide range of foods as soon as they start eating solids.

The French even have a phrase for this: *l'éducation du goût* (the education of taste). And they speak rather poetically about the "*debut de la diversification*" (beginning of food diversification), with the same emotion that parents in many cultures reserve for the moment when their child starts school or takes their first step. When a child starts eating solid foods, they're starting a long and interesting journey. Quite the contrast to the dull, prosaic English equivalent: "starting solid foods"!

How does early food diversification work, practically speaking? Take the case of Hélène, the French mom living in LA. When she started her son Pablo on solid foods, she started with vegetable purées. Why veggies first? Delaying fruit for at least a month, so babies get used to the less-sweet taste of vegetables, is a standard recommendation of French pediatricians. Not all French parents follow this rule, but it seems to make sense to include as many veggies as fruits in your baby's menu. Hélène introduced the following vegetables, one after the other, waiting a day or so between each to see if Pablo had any signs of allergic reactions (he didn't). By the age of 8 months, here's what Pablo was eating:

Asparagus (green), steamed with a bit of potato and puréed

Beans (green), steamed and puréed

Broccoli, steamed and puréed

Brussels sprouts, boiled (so they're less bitter, not steamed) with a bit of potato and puréed

Carrots, steamed and puréed

Cauliflower, steamed and puréed

Celery root, steamed with a bit of potato and puréed

Cucumber, steamed with a bit of potato and puréed

Endive, steamed with a bit of potato and puréed

Kale/all chards, steamed with a bit of potato and puréed

Peas, steamed and puréed

Sweet potato, steamed and puréed

Watercress, steamed with a bit of potato and puréed

White leeks, steamed with a bit of potato and puréed (only the top white part of the leek)

Winter squash, steamed and puréed

Zucchini, steamed with a bit of potato and puréed

This is quite the list! But it's not out of the ordinary for French parents. In practice, French parents introduce a new vegetable every few days. A recent study found that they introduced, on average, 6 new veggies in the first month of solid foods, and nearly half the babies in the study were introduced to between 7 and 12 veggies in the first month.[10] French mothers also rotated vegetables on a daily and weekly basis: they made, on average, 18 changes to the way in which they prepared the vegetables offered (some made as many as 27 changes!). The result? French babies are eating—and enjoying—a much greater variety of foods by time they're 2 years old—just when the picky eating phase hits. By the time they are school-age, most have gotten over the picky eating phase. Of course, they're still learning to like a broader variety of foods, but few are on the "beige food" diet that's common in North America.

The list of "first food" vegetables recommended by the French Society of Pediatrics (FSP) might surprise a lot of parents. According to their official baby-feeding guide, babies as young as 5 or 6 months can be introduced to all of the following (in any order) as smooth purées (any of which can be mixed into a small amount of potato, which should be introduced separately first, just as Hélène did): carrots, green beans, spinach, zucchini (peeled and seeds removed), leeks (whites only), pumpkin, baby endive and baby chard (in limited quantities), and green peas (only if they are "extra-fine" and served in small quantities; the French think that green peas are really hard on the digestive system and don't tend to serve them until the babies are a bit older). French pediatricians think these veggies are easy to digest and suitable from 6 months onwards.

If you think that sounds impressive, you'll be even more impressed by the vegetables the FSP recommends introducing from 9 months onward: cabbage, turnip, onion, celery, celery root (celeriac), green peas, tomatoes, Jerusalem artichoke, cardoons, artichoke, peppers, eggplant, and parsley. If these are handled well, then it's on to other veggies, including fennel, cauliflower, broccoli, and beets. (Hélène appears to have jumped the gun on some of these.) Any of these vegetables can now be combined with fish. Indeed, 9-month-old Pablo was eating purée combinations ranging from sole and cucumber to salmon and sorrel to cod and chard! The purées at this age are slightly thicker or may have small lumps or be combined with small pieces of pasta (such as orzo).

Once meat options are introduced, the meals become even more interesting. By the time he was a year old, Pablo was eating chicken *jardinière* (with carrot, turnip, green beans, and flat-leaf parsley), veal and green asparagus (tips only), and (my personal favorite) lamb and rutabaga purée (by this time a lumpier dish with small, chewable morsels). Pablo had also transitioned to finger foods.

Here's one of Pablo's sample daily menus from when he was 13 months old. Note: both lunch and dinner follow the traditional four-course meal structure: appetizer, main course, cheese course, dessert.

Breakfast
Baby oatmeal with milk
Fruit (berries)
Plain Greek yogurt with a sprinkle of wheat germ
Orange juice

Lunch
Appetizer/finger foods: Greek salad (grated cucumber, tomatoes, feta cheese)
Main course: Boeuf ratatouille purée
Cheese: Gouda
Dessert: Yogurt and fresh apricot slices

Snack
Apple-pear compote

Dinner

Appetizer/finger foods: Endive and green bean salad with
blue cheese

Main course: Roasted pork ribs (small pieces from his
parents' servings), herbed broccoli purée

Cheese: Petit Basque sheep's milk cheese

Dessert: Plain Greek yogurt

On his 18-month "birthday," Pablo's lunch menu looked like
this:

Appetizer/finger foods: Cold (cooked) zucchini, mint, and
feta salad

Main course: Veal liver with green beans (with garlic and
flat-leaf parsley)

Cheese: Creamy Italian blue cheese

Dessert: Plain yogurt with fresh fruit

For his afternoon snack, Pablo ate persimmon seeds; dinner
included roasted butternut squash and coconut soup, Dover sole
fillets with quinoa, and Camembert! Hélène explains that Pablo
is simply eating what the adults are eating, appropriately adapted
(for example, his fish is cut up carefully to make sure there are no
bones). Indeed, from 18 months onward, the FSP suggests that
babies can eat nearly everything adults eat (although they recommend waiting on dried beans such as kidney beans until they
can chew them properly, otherwise they present a choking
hazard).

When *New York Times* reporter Keith Dixon tried this with
his 8-month-old daughter, Gracie, he was pleasantly surprised
by the results. With the help of a food mill, little Gracie happily devoured ravioli with sage butter, pecorino, and crispy
sage leaves. Mashing up cannellini beans with rosemary oil and
shallots proved to be a winner, too. Keith and his wife tried
giving Gracie pretty much anything they were eating: lentils
milled with caramelized onions and wilted rocket or flaked white

fish, stirring in ripe, fresh fruits (such as pears) or water or healthy oils (such as flax oil) to achieve a nice consistency. Keith even verified this approach with Dr. Bhatia, who liked the meal-sharing idea, as feeding a baby a range of foods encourages them to be more adventurous at the table.[11]

This approach might not get everyone's approval. In fact, the American Academy of Pediatrics (AAP) warns parents against foods like spinach and against some home-prepared baby foods:

If you make your own baby food, be aware that home-prepared spinach, beets, green beans, squash, and carrots are not good choices during early infancy. They may contain large amounts of nitrates. Nitrates are chemicals that can cause an unusual type of anemia (low blood count) in young babies. Commercially prepared vegetables are safer because the manufacturers test for nitrates. Peas, corn, and sweet potatoes are better choices for home-prepared baby foods.[12]

The AAP guidelines are very cautious, particularly about vegetables. The first food they mention on their HealthyChild.org website is baby cereal. They do mention some vegetables (squash, peas, corn, carrots), but don't provide a specific list (and don't divide this list into age categories). When they provide a sample daily menu for an 8- to 12-month-old baby, they simply mention "yellow or orange vegetables" and "green vegetables." Not specific enough to be helpful, in my opinion. And what about red vegetables, or purple ones?

In short, the advice from French and American pediatricians is contradictory, and American pediatricians don't agree with each other on the best approach to feeding babies. (The official AAP advice contradicts that of the FSP as well as Dr. Bhatia's views, even though he is a member of the AAP committee on nutrition!) Confusing, I know. But comparing the two approaches suggests you can probably be more ambitious about food diversification than the American guidelines suggest. My recommendation: do your own research and talk to your health-care provider about what makes sense for your family. Your health-care provider will also be able to give you the most up-to-date advice on allergies and on foods that you should delay introducing, such as eggs, shellfish, unpasteurized honey, nuts, and citrus.

Whatever first foods you *do* serve to your baby, remember that many doctors still recommend waiting a day after introducing each one to see if there are any allergic reactions. By the time they're 9 months old, babies should be able to start eating the purée recipes that begin on page 211. If you add those in progressively, your child will be eating a broad range of vegetables by the time they are 2 years old.

It's worth noting that some researchers and pediatricians are increasingly questioning the North American approach to child feeding, particularly the emphasis on a limited variety of foods in the first year and the choice of processed white rice cereal as the first food for babies. Dr. David Ludwig, Director of the Optimal Weight for Life Program at the Boston Children's Hospital (a leading obesity research center), argues that conventional white rice baby cereal—which has had most of the vitamins and nutrients removed through processing—is the nutritional equivalent of table sugar.[13] He argues that such foods raise blood sugar and insulin levels without providing nutrients (apart from the added iron).[14] In other words, rice cereal might just be among the worst foods for infants.

How is it possible that something so nutritionally bankrupt became a cornerstone of our infant diet? It may be because some rice cereals are iron-fortified, and iron is one of the few widespread nutritional deficiencies in the United States.[15] However, there are other ways to provide iron, notably through naturally iron-rich foods (like spinach), provided they are served with a little vitamin C (found in tomatoes, for example) to help with absorption.

Are the infant and child feeding guidelines currently recommended in North America, which often lead to children receiving the bulk of calories in the form of heavily processed rice cereal and other carbs, inadvertently training children to prefer processed and junk food?[16] Some doctors think so. Well-known pediatrician Dr. Alan Greene argues that this approach teaches children to prefer certain kinds of foods such as white bread, crackers, and pasta.[17] By 18 months, few American toddlers are eating whole grains on a daily basis. Dr. Greene encourages parents to serve brown rice cereals instead (or homemade rice mash or vegetable purée) and has even launched a "WhiteOut Campaign" calling for an end to the recommendation of serving processed cereals—specifically white rice cereal—to babies (drgreene.com/whiteout). It may make sense to think twice about rice cereal.

When should I start taste training my baby?

As soon as your baby starts eating solid foods! It's relatively easy at this stage since most babies are naturally curious about new foods (just as they are with new toys). In fact, most babies will put everything into their mouths, food and non-food items (my older daughter even sampled rocks, gravel, and dirt!)[18] Take advantage of their natural curiosity to get them sampling lots of different tastes—and not just bland tastes!

Recommendations for when to start solid foods vary between countries and when the recommendations were written. At the moment, 6 months seems to be the preferred age (introducing solid foods before the age of 4 months may raise the risk of allergies). Pediatric recommendations in some countries also suggest avoiding some foods (such as unpasteurized honey) until 12 months or older. Check the guidelines that are relevant for you, then consult with your pediatrician and specifically discuss any foods that may pose allergy risks for your child. Whenever you start, your goal should be to take advantage of your baby's natural curiosity about foods and to introduce lots of variety before they are 2 years old, when the picky eating phase begins for many children.

You should know, however, that there is no magical age at which babies are ready. Some babies will be interested earlier, some not. My first daughter was tremendously interested in food at the age of 4 months. My second daughter wasn't interested until later, and since she didn't have many teeth until quite late, she was slow to start chewing solid foods.

Each baby develops differently—your baby will be your best guide. They will let you know when they are ready! Some babies may mimic you eating, bringing their hand up to their faces. Others may grunt or gesture, and even try reaching for the food. When they do start eating, some babies may have trouble keeping the food in their mouths. At this age, their natural extrusion reflex may cause them to push food out of their mouth with their tongue. This natural protective mechanism will disappear after a few weeks or months at most.

Stick to simple, single-ingredient dishes for the first month or two, after which you can try introducing fun combinations. Babies can start eating herbs and spices at 9 months, which is why the purée recipes in the second part of this book contain ingredients like cinnamon, oregano, cumin, and basil. *Yum!*

Do I need any special equipment?

In terms of gear, I personally believe less is more. At a minimum, you'll probably find it helpful to have a high chair, an unbreakable baby spoon and bowl, bibs, and at least one device for puréeing food, whether it be a food mill, food processor or blender. A BebeCook machine steams and purées all at once, and can even defrost! You can achieve the same results (and smoother purées) with a simple steamer insert for one of your pots and a blender.

When and how do I feed my baby?

There is no magic formula or one-size-fits-all rule to teaching your child to be a good eater, but the following are some tips that will work for most families.

Do **create a schedule.** It can be fluid and flexible, but create some notion of a schedule that includes three meals a day served roughly at the same times as your meals. Add scheduled snacks as appropriate. The FSP recommends one snack per day (in the mid-afternoon), whereas the AAP recommends three (mid-morning, mid-afternoon, and bedtime). A simple daily schedule might look like this: breakfast between 8 and 9 a.m., lunch between 12 and 1 p.m., snack at 3:30 p.m., and dinner between 5:30 and 6:30 p.m. Naptimes, illnesses, playdates, and other commitments will of course mean that you'll vary these times a bit. Not to worry! Whatever schedule you adopt, the point is to clearly distinguish eating times from non-eating times.

Don't **try to control your baby's eating.** It's your job to schedule meals and to present a good variety of food in a relaxed, comfortable setting. It's your baby's job to decide whether and how much they eat. Don't insist that they eat more if they're full, don't insist that they eat things they're refusing, and, above all, never force your baby to eat.

Do **watch out for choking hazards, and for hot spots when rewarming food.** Puréed foods are best for younger babies, and chewable foods, which are generally introduced between 10 and 12 months, should be offered cautiously at first. When transitioning babies to chewable foods, make sure the dishes are cooked until they can be easily squashed with a fork. Make bite sizes teeny-tiny (about the size of a raisin). An easy rule of thumb: any food placed in the child's mouth should be able to be swallowed as is, without chewing.

Do **make variety a habit by rotating through foods regularly.** If babies get used to novelty early on, they're less likely to develop a restricted favorite foods list as toddlers (only pancakes for breakfast, only pasta for lunch, and so on). Introduce as much variety as you can, in colors as well as flavors. Establish the expectation that novelty is normal.

Don't **worry if your baby makes a mess.** Of course babies will sometimes make a mess. How much mess you are willing to tolerate is up to you, but it's not a concern. If you do want your baby to eat tidily, it's certainly possible. Watching French babies taught me that babies can actually learn to eat relatively tidily, right from the start. For starters, they simply aren't allowed to play with their food! For example, throwing food means that the plate is removed (once and for all!) from the table, and even young babies quickly learn that if they're hungry they'd better not throw their carrot purée at the floor.

Do **make homemade baby food.** This can be fast and easy if you're organized. Freezing purées in large batches saves time, and you can also mix homemade with store-bought purées to introduce more taste variety. Committing to make homemade purées means that you'll have lots of fruits and veggies around—and eat more of them yourself, too. If you're worried about time not spent with your baby, put them in their high chair in the middle of the kitchen and give them some pots and pans and spoons to bang and play with. They'll have fun watching you and "cooking," too!

Do **eat everything your baby eats!** Research shows that children are much more likely to try a new food if their parent tries it first—with obvious enjoyment. If it isn't tasty for you, then it might not be for your baby, either. Try new combinations; sometimes your baby may be ready for more interesting tastes, which will sustain their interest in foods.

Don't **add extra salt to baby's food.** If you're serving your baby a portion of an adult dish, make sure to remove their portion before you add salt. Remember that babies have on average many more taste buds than adults. They'll enjoy the natural flavors without the salt.

Do **steam veggies whenever possible.** For meats and fish, any cooking method that retains moisture (such as poaching fish) is a good bet, as this will make it easier for babies to chew and swallow.

Do **vary your cooking methods in order to give some taste variety.** Steaming is best in terms of nutrient conservation, but you can also sauté in a little butter, olive oil, or canola oil (sautéed zucchini is delicious, for example, as are red peppers). Roasting is easy but time-consuming, and will intensify flavors (especially of squash and sweet potatoes). Roasting also allows you to prepare combinations of adult and baby veggies at the same time—just cut the veggies in large chunks, add water, and roast in the oven at 190°C/gas 5 until tender. Season and serve your portion, and purée your baby's portion. *Voila!*

Don't **get stuck in a rut.** When making food combinations for your purées, don't be afraid to vary the quantities of the base ingredients. If the purée tastes slightly different each time, so much the better! Your baby will get used to more novelty.

Do **offer finger foods as your child develops the "pincer grip" between forefinger and thumb some time between 10 and 12 months old.** Be sure to slice any smooth foods (such as grapes or cherry tomatoes) into small pieces to avoid choking hazards. Small pieces of chopped-up veggies (such as green peas) or fruit (such as blueberries) make for great finger foods.

Don't **be averse to a little fat in your child's food.** Children need to eat a moderate amount of healthy fats for optimum growth and development. Fat helps with the absorption of fat-soluble nutrients. Plus, fat adds flavor! A dab of butter on spinach purée will make it that much more palatable. You can also use high-quality oils (such as olive oil) in moderation.

Do **have your child sit at the table while eating.** It's a good habit, if only for safety reasons: kids are less likely to choke when sitting calmly and focusing on chewing.

Do **eat yourself at baby's mealtime.** Babies are natural mimics, and it's an educational experience for them to sit with you at the table. As they see their older siblings and parents or caregivers trying new foods, they'll be more likely to try new things.[19]

Do **keep a diary of what your child is eating and their reactions.** It will help you think about what to introduce next and remind you about including variety, plus you'll be able to see emerging patterns of likes and dislikes.

Don't **allow emphatic expressions of food dislikes at your family table.** Children are highly suggestible; if another child or adult declares that he or she doesn't like something, chances are your baby will follow suit. Teach your other family members to either say nothing or to politely say "no, thank you."[20]

Don't **assume your baby won't like something.** Let them decide. If it's safe to eat, let them try it. And don't assume their food preferences will be like yours. That being said, your child will refuse to try foods, so prepare yourself for the inevitable.

What do I do when my baby refuses to try a new food?

Food refusals are one of the most frustrating aspects of parenting. They raise our anxiety levels and often feel like rejection. The most important thing (and I know this is hard to do): don't pressure your baby in any way. Simply remove the food without comment and do not offer a replacement or substitute. You don't want to fall into the trap of short-order cooking, and you don't want to reinforce the refusal behavior. Try offering the food again in a few days or a few weeks.

Feeding your baby is like a conversation. If you're sensitive to their cues, your baby will gain confidence. You'll avoid creating emotional associations with food, and your baby will learn the skill of eating at their own pace.

Remember that babies are acute tasters. They have more taste buds on average than adults. Babies can distinguish different kinds of sugars from one another—even at low concentrations.[21] They can even distinguish their mother's breast milk from another's breast milk just a few days after being born! They are highly capable of tasting and enjoying the full range of flavors in all foods—all the more reason not to give them solely bland food (but it may take them a few tries to get used to it).

Following the vegetable rotation rule will help you deal with food refusals as well. Rotating vegetables frequently keeps things interesting (and later on, with toddlers, lowers tension at the table, particularly if you make sure your child is being served foods they like in between the "scary" foods)! Of course, if you offer greater variety, you will find more things that your child does like, and you'll be less likely to create a battle of wills over foods that kids don't like (see page 119).[22] Remember, learning to like vegetables is a matter of "practice makes perfect."

Another point to remember is that while each baby has their own distinct eating style, there are common developmental patterns most babies share. Most babies between the ages of 2 and 3 will show more negative reactions to food, become more distractible when eating (sound familiar?), before they eventually develop more predictable appetite patterns over time.[23] The emergence of negative food reactions is thought to be a normal developmental pattern, as babies start figuring out what they like (and don't like) and as their diet becomes more varied and diverse.[24] Distractibility increases as children reach the age of 2, when their growth slows down and their appetite diminishes.[25] Around this time, you'll probably also notice that your baby's appetite will become increasingly predictable (with regular times when they are hungry), as their eating style becomes apparent and as they start to adapt to your family's eating schedule.

At the same time, you'll start to learn more about your baby's individual eating style, which is evident even in babies as young as 6 months.[26] Babies (just like adults) tend to exhibit one of three eating styles:

1. **The Easy Eater.** This type of eater (about 3 in 10 babies) has a more predictable appetite and is less distractible at mealtimes—basically, they're really interested in food, eager to get it, and won't let much get in their way if they're hungry. They're not fussy, usually calm at mealtimes, and generally open to new food experiences. Often, these children also have a low emotional reactivity; they're the easy-going kids. My nephew Damien is this type of eater; he'll focus with single-minded intensity on getting the most food in as little time as possible. With Damien (as is sometimes the case with kids in this category), overeating is occasionally a concern.

2. **The Strong-minded Eater.** This type of eater has a fairly predictable appetite, is somewhat (but not too) distractible at mealtimes, and has clear food preferences: likes and dislikes that emerge early and may intensify over time. This type of eater (approximately 5 or 6 out of 10 babies) is sometimes a handful, and sometimes reacts to new foods, but generally gets used to them over time. My younger daughter, Claire, is this type of eater—mostly happy to eat, but not afraid to express her likes and dislikes.

3. **The Reactive Eater.** These children (approximately 1 or 2 out of 10 babies) react very strongly to foods and tend to have a narrow set of preferred foods. They're often more distractible at mealtimes and have a less predictable appetite pattern; they may also be more anxious about eating and more emotionally reactive to food (and to things in general). These children are the most likely to be strongly neophobic (afraid of new foods) when they are toddlers, and it will take more time and persistence to help them learn to eat a varied diet. If this describes your child, I can empathize: my older daughter, Sophie, was a reactive eater. The days of her "crazy food dance" (in

which she would roll her eyes, stamp her feet, and even jump up and down if presented with a food she didn't like) are long gone, but none of us had an easy time.[27] With Sophie, as is sometimes the case with fussy eaters, getting her to eat enough food was sometimes a worry. (How long can a toddler survive on smoothies and buttered toast?)

Your baby has their own "eating personality" with traits as durable and long-lasting as other aspects of their personality. Your job is to figure out your child's eating style and encourage them to expand their palate while being respectful of their individual differences. Some babies will go more slowly than others, but don't give up hope! You *can* teach your child to eat—with the right combination of love and limits, persistence and perspective, encouragement and common sense.

Toddlers: Preventing and Solving Common Eating Challenges

Feeding toddlers and preschoolers is often frustrating. Anxious to make sure their children are getting enough nutritious food, parents are often confronted with children with strong taste preferences who want to eat the same foods nearly every day (often the more unhealthy foods in the family repertoire).

Parents know what to feed their toddlers (usually, more fruits and vegetables), but they don't know *how* to get them to eat those healthy things. Many toddlers prefer bland foods (things made with white refined flour, such as crackers and bread) to anything else. I know this from personal experience: when she was 2, my oldest daughter would have eaten nothing but pasta and buttered toast if we'd let her. Many of my test families reported something similar. This, of course, is developmentally normal: whereas babies are exploring yet closely attached, toddlers are becoming little individuals—at times resisting parents while exploring their individuality and new-found sense of power.

As a result, few toddlers and preschoolers eat the recommended five servings of fruits and vegetables a day. Their eating patterns are often unpredictable; sometimes they seem very hungry; other times they seem completely uninterested in food. The USDA recommendation that *half* your plate should be fruits and vegetables (at every meal!) can seem almost laughable when confronted with the fickle, finicky tastes of younger children.

Despite all of this, my main message is still *don't worry*. If your child's height and weight are within the normal range according to your health-care provider, and if your child looks healthy and is usually happy and full of energy, then their picky eating behaviors are likely just a normal phase of development. There are, however, some warning signs to look out for. If your child seems to have trouble chewing, regularly refuses most foods, does not have regular bowel movements that are soft and easy to pass at least once every day or two, urinates less than four times per day, is not sleeping 10 to 12 hours per night, and is not eating at least one item from each of the main food groups—fruits, vegetables, grains, proteins (such as meat, fish, beans, nuts, and seeds), dairy (or substitutes), and healthy fats and oils—a day, then you should consult your health-care practitioner.

In most cases, your child's picky eating habits are likely to be completely normal. Your worries about your child's eating habits are also normal. Many parents are concerned that their child eats too many unhealthy foods (such as refined white flour, sugar, processed foods), doesn't eat enough healthy foods (vegetables, proteins, and whole grains typically feature high on this list), or simply doesn't eat enough, period. You're not alone! Picky eating is a developmental phase, and most children will need your guidance in order to overcome it. Remember: you can teach a child to eat just like you teach them to read—but they do need regular practice and your guidance.

Creating healthy boundaries—using the simple routines and rules introduced in the Seven Secrets—is an important part of this guidance. *How* and *when* kids eat (for example, with a structured routine of three meals and one or two snacks per day) helps with *what* kids eat. Remember your routine, and stick to it.

Remember those routines!

The toddler years are the best time to establish healthy eating practices. Some suggestions include:

- Schedule meals and snacks (and stick to it).
- Eat at the table and nowhere else (no chasing a distractible toddler around the house with a spoon and a bowl—if for no other reason than it's a choking hazard).
- Avoid pressure at the table: no catering, forcing, bribing, cajoling, enticing.
- Kids eat what adults eat: no short-order cooking and no substitutes.
- Follow the "variety" rule: introduce one new food per day (or per week or whatever time period suits your family). Trust me: novelty will work for you rather than against you. This is your way of giving your toddler the opportunity to learn to eat new foods.
- Follow the "rotation" rule: serve old favorites in new ways, every single day.
- Parents provide, kids decide: be appropriately encouraging about tasting new foods, but let your toddler decide what they do and don't eat.
- Create rituals: table talk rituals, politeness rules—if you instil them now, it will be much, much easier when they're older. Really!

Establishing routines like these sets the stage for learning new tastes and textures: your toddler will come to meals hungry, in a positive mindset, and ready to behave reasonably well when at the table.

Another important strategy is to adapt your meals slightly (just ever so slightly) to your toddler's developing eating abilities. Here are some key tips:

- Make sure your child is comfy: feet propped up and with good back support. Believe it or not, toddlers' chewing effectiveness depends on how well their core is supported—by their feet! Prop up their feet with firm support.
- Make food physically easy to eat (meat is soft and moist; salad is cut up as finger food).
- Serve small servings: allow your child to ask for more, but don't serve them too much at the start.
- Serve veggies or fruit first, preferably at both lunch and dinner.

A little cautionary note: the rules and routines aren't meant to make mealtimes overly rigid. Toddlers learn to eat best when their parents are relaxed. If you start early enough and are persistent enough, by the time your child is school-age (around 6 years old), they'll be eating more or less like an adult. You'll have introduced a range of textures and tastes into your child's diet and helped them learn a structured eating routine. Food will increasingly be a source of fun for the whole family (and not a cause for food fights).

Along the way, though, you're likely to encounter three challenges. Many toddlers have difficulty:

1. accepting different textures
2. mixing foods (and eating "mixed" dishes)
3. interpreting and coordinating signals from different senses (sight, hearing, touch, smell, and taste) when encountering new foods.

Below are some simple tips and tricks to help you overcome these challenges.

The toddler texture challenge

Toddlerhood is the stage when children begin encountering—and mastering—different textures. Chewing seems so natural to adults that it is easy to forget this is a big step up from babyhood. Think of how difficult it must be to learn to like crunching hard foods. I still have a very clear memory of how proud my older daughter was when she first munched through a raw carrot—no mean feat, given those little teeth and that little jaw!

Discomfort with textures is a common problem for toddlers, and it's often an important reason they enjoy (or reject) foods.[1] Part of the reason is mechanical: toddlers' teeth and jaws (as well as the surrounding muscles) are still developing, and so it may be difficult for them to be in full control of certain foods in their mouths.[2] Toddlers will tend to reject textures that are difficult to manipulate in their mouths (and rightly so, from their perspective!). Vegetables, with their slippery, slimy textures (like mushrooms) or hard, crunchy textures (which some kids find difficult), or (even worse) combined soft and slippery textures (raw tomatoes), are literally hard for kids to get their teeth into.[3]

Toddler suspicion of textures is thus at least partially a natural protective mechanism against the risk of choking. Although choking is indeed a risk (see below), you'll want to help your child figure out which textures they *can* eat without risk. The texture play aspect of the games and experiments listed here will help you do just that.

The simplest approach of all is to adapt the textures of the foods you are serving to suit your toddler's evolving skills. Here are some examples:

- If your child is starting to learn to eat lettuce, try ripping it into very small pieces or serving only the hard spine of the lettuce leaves, which is crunchier and more like the apples, carrots, and celery they might already be enjoying.
- Make sure that any meat you serve is cut into very

small morsels and is seriously tender and moist. Often, an aversion to meat is a rejection of texture (and the demands of chewing), not taste. See page 196 for tips.

- Turn texture into a game in its own right. In our house, we invented the Carrot Crunch variation of Game 13: Terrific Textures (page 123) to encourage our younger daughter to eat crunchy carrots. Preschoolers are playful and love to imitate parents. Take advantage of those tendencies!

Gagging versus choking

Gagging is a normal reflex that helps to prevent choking: when food slips to the back of the mouth, gagging pushes it forward again. Knowing that, try to remember that if you don't react to your child gagging, they won't either. They'll continue eating. Just calmly explain that gagging is no reason to worry, and teach them how to avoid it by taking small mouthfuls and chewing properly.

Choking is, of course, dangerous. If a child is able to breathe, or cough, they will probably expel the food item themselves. But if a child is making no sound or only a squeaky, whistling sound, they may be choking. Choking tends to happen when you breathe in at the same time you swallow. The risk is higher with slippery foods (such as hot dogs, sausages, grapes, baby carrots—foods that are just the right size to clog up the windpipe) and with foods that are tough to chew (such as steak, hard nuts, or candies) or sticky (such as large globs of peanut butter). Make sure to protect your child by avoiding the above-mentioned foods before the age of 3 and chopping up foods after that age (for instance, cut grapes into quarters). Encourage your child to be calm at the table and to eat only when seated. Most important, have your health-care provider teach you basic first aid for choking.

Mixing textures

Many children don't like mixing different textured foods together. This is completely normal and a passing phase. Part of the reason is simply that toddlers are still learning to chew and manipulate foods in their mouths, and mixing textures makes this more complicated. Another reason is that kids are still learning (and shuffling) cognitive categories at this age. For example, if you serve carrots in a slightly different way (say, sprinkled with parsley rather than the plain style they're used to), kids may see this as an entirely new dish. This is why they're sometimes happy to eat certain foods on their own, but not mixed together. A classic example: 3-year-old Tobias, the son of one of my test families, liked red peppers and scrambled eggs, but serve him an omelet with red peppers in it and he'd refuse to eat it.

The solution? Put your child in charge, as my test families did, with great results:

Tobias doesn't like things combined ... unless he gets to mix them himself. I think it gives him a sense of control, because I've noticed that if he gets to do the mixing, there's no problem. So if I'm introducing him to a new food, I now get him to help me make the dish. We made an omelet together last week, which was an experiment because he doesn't really like omelets (although he's actually really good at breaking eggs and can crack them single-handed without getting any shells in the bowl!). We added peppers and spinach and lots of cheese, and we watched it all bubble up together. It was so nice, for both of us. This was after a long day of work, so cooking together served as quality time as well as my time to make dinner. And he ate it and said it was delicious. Sometimes for lunch or on lazy evenings I give him a piece of pita bread and let him fill it with cucumbers and cheese or leftover chicken or steak— so as long as he's doing the adding, he's fine with it.

—Martha

Three-year-old Tobias's experience is typical of many kids his age. Different textures combined in a single dish are often challenging for young children. But you can help your child get over this fear! Game 16: The Mixing Game (page 144 develops this idea into a set of sequenced games that will help your child get used to the idea of mixing textures.

Taste and texture testing

The toddler stage is when the taste-testing approach becomes your best friend. For cautious toddlers, visual exposure *prior* to taste testing can have really positive effects. This might include showing a vegetable, fruit, or dish to your child, allowing them to handle the ingredients, or reading books about food out loud (some great children's books with positive messages about food are listed on GettingToYum.com.

Remember: you can use taste testing to explore textures as well as tastes. If you think you're too busy to organize taste testing, try incorporating it into your daily cooking routine. Before you mash the potatoes, set one aside; serve a slice of boiled potato along with the mashed potatoes and ask your child to compare the two. Or use the "rotation" rule to help you explore textures: serve carrots raw one day, parboiled the next, in a soup the day after! Taste testing isn't complicated or time-consuming, but it does require you to be attentive and a little inventive. Above all, try to avoid "sneaky chef" strategies. They're nutritionally okay, but developmentally questionable. Keep offering your child opportunities to learn to eat the "scary foods"—the more frequently (and calmly) you do so, the more quickly they'll come around.

The games your toddler might play with you

Toddlers love to test boundaries and push buttons, and are just beginning to explore what power struggles are all about. They're really like little psychologists, trying to figure out what they can get away with and whether they can get a reaction (happiness, anger, fear, annoyance) out of others. This experimentation is normal, but can also be scary for toddlers. They do want firm boundaries and will respond well when these are in place, as Hélène, mother of 18-month-old Pablo, found out:

A recent challenge was when Pablo discovered one of his many superpowers: taking off his bib in the middle of the meal. I had originally established a rule that we must wear a bib and sit in the high chair to eat. When he discovered I was annoyed when he was taking off his bib, he started doing it repeatedly, very early in the meal, and would push me into a power struggle. I fell in that trap a couple of times and then realized my error. A power struggle was making the situation worse, and it was ruining my meal, as I would get upset. And he wouldn't eat any more anyway. So I thought, okay, just go with a simple, calm consequence.

The next time he took off his bib mid-meal, I said nonchalantly, "Okay, you are done with eating? Fine by me." (I was thinking to myself, if he's hungry, he'll eat better at the next meal.) And I let him leave the table, while we continued to eat our meal. The first couple of times I did this, he was pretty surprised and hung out near us, trying to get our attention. After about four times, he stopped taking off his bib during the meal. Now, at the end of the meal, he points to it, saying "Maman" with his sweet voice and signing "please," to ask if he can take off his bib. I ask him if he's finished eating, and if he's not, we go on with the meal. If he is, so be it. I was relieved this worked!

—*Hélène*

Remember: children may decide to test your rules and routines, particularly if you are implementing them when they're a bit older. A child may decide to misbehave at the table; if so, you might have to ask them to leave and be firm about them not coming back to finish the meal or be with the family, explaining that they can try again at the next meal. A toddler may repeatedly try to remove their bib; if so, firmly signal that the meal is over. If you're firm, they'll quickly learn.

A common way young children will test boundaries is the "I won't eat" tactic. My younger daughter tried this on us when she wasn't quite 3 years old. "I *won't* eat," she announced one dinnertime. "Fine," we said. "It's bedtime, so you can go upstairs and go to bed." "*Fine!*" she huffed and dramatically stormed (well, as much as a 3-year-old can storm) up to her bedroom. We said nothing and happily continued on with our meal. Within 5 minutes, she had come back to the table, settled in, and started eating. We didn't make a big deal of it, and it never happened again.

A variation on the previous tactic is the "I'm not hungry" strategy. It may very well be that your child is not hungry (did they have a big piece of cake at a birthday party in the late afternoon?), but they also may just be pushing your buttons. Here's one approach that Ellyn Satter, a doyenne of American nutrition writers, recommends: simply say, "You don't have to eat, but come and keep us company for a few minutes." If they choose to leave: "Fine, but that is all until your next mealtime." If they come back to the table to eat, let them do so without much comment. If they fuss, don't get angry (you're paying them attention, and thus rewarding them). If you're firm, your child will probably only try this gambit on you once.

Other strategies have been covered in earlier chapters:

- **"I don't like that!"** The "veggies first" and "you just have to taste it" rules help you deal with the inevitable "I don't like that" responses.
- **"I want pasta!"** Remember, you've committed to avoiding short-order cooking, so no pasta (or whatever else they may be demanding) on short notice if they don't like what they see on the table. It's exhausting for you and doesn't offer opportunities for your child to learn. At our house we like the

motto "You get what you get, and you don't get upset." Make sure there is something they like on the table (like bread) that they can eat if they really don't want to eat anything else.

- **"Look at me, Mommy!"** A more subtle game sometimes revolves around praise: children exaggerate good (or alternate good and bad) behavior in order to get praise from adults. A simple way to avoid this is to not give excessive praise. You can comment if they eat well, but don't go over the top, and don't praise for behavior that's ordinary (or should be ordinary). The important thing is that *they* are proud of themselves; it's not *your* issue. The dinner-table conversation should not revolve around your child's eating habits; as explored in Secret 4: Routines and Rituals Make Healthy Eating Automatic (and Fun!) (page 89), there are other "table talk" strategies that you can use.

Keep it positive! Balancing love and limits

Toddlers have a lot to learn about eating, and there's a lot to remember as a parent. Ultimately, it's all about striking a healthy balance between love and limits. At times, you'll want to be firmer; at other times, try a lighter touch. In general, you're probably being too controlling if you make your child clean their plate, eat all of their food before dessert, stay at the table (after everyone has left) to finish their food, or only let them eat three meals a day (kids do need at least one snack). On the other hand, you're probably not setting strong enough limits if you short-order cook or produce special food for your child at many meals, let your child have snacks (or juice or milk) whenever they want, allow your child to behave badly at the table, or bribe your child with food to do basic tasks. Creating good routines now will serve you well for a lifetime.

School-Age Children: Smart Strategies for Raising Food-Savvy Kids

Raising healthy eaters takes a different turn when your children are school-age. They're now spending more time in environments beyond parental control, exposed to the pressures of school food offerings and peers. The landscape they're negotiating is much more complex—luckily, they're old enough to start learning the skills they need. And they do need to learn them in order to develop the autonomy they need as adults.

As explored in Secret 2: Marketing Healthy Food to Your Kids Really Works!, children need the ability to decipher the marketing messages they encounter everywhere around them—particularly on TV and online, but also at school.[1] The American Academy of Pediatrics (AAP) recommends no screen time for kids under the age of 2, and only 1 to 2 hours per day for older kids (the average is 4 hours per day).[2]

An equally powerful strategy to limiting exposure is counter-marketing, which provides your kids with the skills to resist marketing messages. Kids have to be aware that ads surround them and be able to identify them. They need to understand what the ads are trying to do, and they need to be motivated to resist the advertising.[3]

As discussed in Secret 2, counter-marketing isn't purely defensive. You can market healthy food to your kids, too! Some of the games and experiments listed in this chapter are designed to help you do "positive marketing" by making healthy food fun and interesting for kids. Sound crazy? Think back to Game 5: The Silly Name Game on page 64. Kids' consumption of vegetables went up by as much as 100 percent when parents and teachers gave playful names to dishes. We do this all the time at our house! Would you rather eat pearl barley or Fairy Baguette? An avocado smoothie or a Monster Smoothie?

For older kids, this is no less important, but your "marketing" techniques—as shown here—will become more subtle. Encourage your tween and adolescent children to develop food preferences and tastes as part of their exploration of individual identity. One of my test family parents, for example, was thrilled that their teenage son discovered a love of green beans; he even ended up cooking them regularly for his family! This is another important point: many teenagers will also develop an interest in cooking food for themselves as part of their journey toward independence.

In addition to marketing, the other key strategy at this age is *modeling* good eating behaviors. Continue with the healthy routines you've already set up (or create them now): three meals and one snack per day. Your older children may seem to need the family meal less (or may even complain about having to join you every day), but they need it just as much as they did when they were younger. They may even enjoy helping you prepare and cook food. In fact, one of the best ways to help a child learn to like new foods is to have them prepare it. They might even be interested in keeping a food discovery diary, or researching fruits and vegetables.

As you model these healthy habits, keep in mind an important goal: helping your child to develop their own informed judgment about food and eating habits. Don't forget that your child is still developing skills. Some children are even continuing to develop fine motor skills by holding cutlery, cutting and moving food from their plates into their mouths. Children also learn to multitask: listening to and participating in a conversation while eating is a valuable skill they'll have for life.

Neither modeling nor marketing imply that you're making all of the decisions for your child. If you're too controlling, your child will likely either completely rebel or depend too much on you to tell them what to do; either way, they won't develop their own judgment. You need to have informed discussions about marketing and the ways in which the manufacturers of processed foods try to manipulate our senses to get us to consume more. Some of the experiments in this chapter help you do just that. But the best way to explore these issues is to discuss them regularly. A regular family meal (whether breakfast or dinner, once a day or once a week) provides the best setting to do that. Building on the lessons, games, and experiments in Secret 5: Kids Don't Need Kids' Food (or going back and doing these, if you're reading this book by the time your children are school-age), will help your children learn sensory awareness and discuss their reactions to food, which helps them understand (and expand) their food preferences.

Remember, school-age children (particularly teenagers) are exploring and experimenting, which is natural and normal for their age. Luckily, their caloric needs are such that they can eat all the nutritious foods they need and still have a little room for some nutritionally marginal foods. If your child happily eats the healthy foods you provide at home while getting occasional treats at friends' houses or through using their allowance to buy snacks, then don't get too worried. Keep the big picture in mind: if they enjoy and eat nutritious foods, and are relatively happy with their body image, and if they're responding well to your parenting combination of love and limits, then they're on the right track. If not, you might need to make some adjustments to your routines, along with trying the experiments and games.

Most important, remember that letting children make their own choices, in an age-appropriate way, is the best way to foster healthy eating habits. Parents who overtly control what their children eat are also more likely to have kids that are external eaters (who eat in response to food cues such as the sight and smell of food, whether or not they're hungry) or emotional eaters (who eat in response to emotional rather than physical needs). These types of eaters are more likely to become obese.[4] More subtly (particularly in the case of girls), children may develop a seesaw love/hate, restrictive/binging eating style in which they frequently suppress feelings of hunger and under-eat, raising the risk of periodic overeating (particularly when they break down and eat a forbidden food).[5]

This doesn't mean that parents shouldn't exert influence on what their children eat. Rather, they need to look for different methods: encouraging, teaching, and modeling (positive), rather than controlling (negative). Research suggests that strategies of covert control, in which parents control the child's food intake in a way that can't directly be detected by a child is a better strategy. At its simplest, this means creating a positive food environment for your child, in which healthy foods are essentially the only choice on a day-to-day basis. This might mean choosing to avoid restaurants that sell unhealthy foods, establishing a "no processed food" rule for grocery shopping, or creating a "once in a while treat" list, but otherwise serving mostly unprocessed foods at home. If these are family routines, then children are less likely to question them. This "covert control" actually increases children's consumption of healthy snacks and is associated with reduced obesity risk.[6]

Even covert control goes only so far. What about when your child is in high school, with McDonald's just around the corner at lunchtime? Hopefully you'll have embraced your child's growing autonomy while shaping their ability to make good food choices. You want to develop what psychologists term a sense of "coherence" about food: a feeling of confidence (which arises through predictable routines and good boundaries) and a mixture of optimism and self-control (which comes through children exercising growing autonomy).[7] This is the fine balance you're trying to strike: parents share a degree of control with kids, which evolves as your child develops.

Older Kids: Top Tips for Turning Picky Eaters into Easy Eaters

1. Create a "new food challenge." Get each child to pick a food they don't like, but that they know one of their friends or family members does like. Ask them (helped by you if necessary) to come up with a recipe for that food item, which they can help prepare and serve to the family. The challenge: to convince the child who originally identified the "yucky" food that they might actually eat it. If that's too complicated, ask each child to pick a food they would like to be able to eat. Serve it different ways, every couple of days over a couple of weeks, and tell them that it will take between 7 and 12 tasting sessions before they probably learn to like it. Just like learning to ride a bicycle, you need practice!

2. Practice the "one family, one meal" rule. Involve your child in creating menus, using ground rules (one fresh veggie every meal), and then stick to it. For example, work out a menu schedule on the weekend. Then, at meals during the week, use the "You don't have to eat it, but you do have to taste it" rule if your child is really being difficult. Use logical consequences (this is not a punishment!): for example, if you don't finish your (small) serving of vegetables, no dessert.

3. Involve your child in planning a meal celebration. Get your child to help pick recipes, shop, cook, and prepare food for a family event (or dinner with guests at your house) during which they receive praise from others (not just you) for doing so.

4. Try positive peer pressure. Does your child have any friends or cousins (or know slightly older kids—that often works wonders!) who eat better and who would come over for a meal at your house to lead by example? Ask your visitor to suggest one of their favorite recipes in advance; if they eat it with gusto, there's a greater chance your child will, too.

5. Try the Crunch a Color game. Check out crunchacolor.com.

6. Create a tasting week. Ask each family member to pick a new food they'd like to learn to eat. Allow them to choose their preferred recipes; interested kids can help buy, prepare, and/or serve the foods to the entire family. Kids will enjoy turning the tables when they pick a food that they know one of their parents doesn't particularly like!

A Final Thought: Get Rid of Guilt!

If you're reading this book, it's because you care about helping your child eat better. Please, put aside any blame you might have. You and your child are simply doing your best, and I hope that this book contains ideas that will help you reach your goals.

Putting aside blame also means removing guilt from the family food equation—for both yourself and your child. Don't label foods as good and bad. Rather, teach your child that there are foods that we eat regularly and foods that we eat occasionally. Equally, don't fall into the trap of forcing your child to eat "bad-tasting" food because it's "good for you." Instead, your goal should be to teach them to love the interesting flavors of all sorts of food.

Think of how your approach to food might change if you adopted this view. How would you teach your child the difference between, say, broccoli and chocolate? You might say this: "Chocolate tastes good. And, of course, broccoli does, too. But chocolate is a 'we eat this once in a while' food, while broccoli is a 'we eat this regularly' food." This approach means that kids don't grow up feeling guilty about liking bad-for-you (but good-tasting) foods, and they run a lower risk of developing unhealthy emotional (craving-indulgence-guilt-deprivation-fueled) eating behaviors later in life. This is really important for all children, but especially for toddlers, who may confuse the "food is bad for you" message with "I'm bad" messages, creating a food–guilt association that's hard to shake.

The simple message is this: try to have a positive rather than punitive attitude to food. Fear (of obesity, of not getting enough nutrients) shouldn't be our primary motivation for eating well. Guilt and anxiety shouldn't be our primary emotional associations around food. Your child isn't learning that we eat healthy food because we *have* to, but rather because we *want* to. That's how they—and your entire family—will develop positive food habits that will last a lifetime.

Here's a reminder of the games you can play with your kids to instill those positive food habits.

The 7 Secrets of Happy Eaters Games

Game	Page number	What the game teaches	Age level
1. The Five Senses	page 39	Taste is influenced by the five senses: sight, touch, hearing, smell, and taste. Kids will better understand their reactions to foods (both ones they like, and ones they don't like!).	4 and up
2. The Five Flavors	page 41	The five different flavors: sweet, salty, sour, bitter, and umami (savory).	4 and up
3. Tasty Taste Buds	page 42	The science behind our taste buds, which are just like muscles: they can be trained!	4 and up
4. The Supertaster Game	page 44	We all experience taste differently. It may take correspondingly more (or less) time to learn to like new foods.	6 and up
5. The Silly Name Game	page 64	Labeling foods can incite kids' enthusiasm for new food.	3 and up
6. The Smell–Taste Experiment	page 65	Smell plays a large part in determining how things taste. Artificial flavors are used to fool our taste buds.	6 and up

Game	Page number	What the game teaches	Age level
7. The Mystery Smell Game	page 67	Smell evokes emotions and memories, and affects our feelings about and perceptions of food.	6 and up
8. The Store Brand Versus Name Brand Blind Taste Test	page 68	Brands influence (and can even fool) our sense of taste.	9 and up
9. The Sour Fruit Game	page 83	Sour is an "interesting" rather than a "yucky" taste.	2 and up
10. The Surprise Sack Game	page 85	Surprise introduces an element of fun to new foods at snack-time.	3 and up
11. The Smiley Face Game	page 103	A simple happy face makes eating more enjoyable.	1 and up
12. The Rose, Thorn, and Bud Game	page 105	A great ritual for keeping kids entertained at the table.	5 and up
13. Terrific Textures	page 123	Textures are more complex when foods are combined. Kids will learn to appreciate "adult" textures.	3 and up
14. The Color Confusion Experiment	page 127	Color influences our sense of taste.	6 and up
15. The Yogurt Game	page 128	Our sense of taste can be fooled by artificial coloring.	6 and up
16. The Mixing Game	page 144	This game teaches your child to enjoy different textures, and to develop their mixing skills, so they'll eat foods with combined textures more easily.	2 and up

Game	Page number	What the game teaches	Age level
17. Make-Your-Own Kids' Salad Game	page 146	This child-led cooking strategy helps kids overcome a common food dislike: salad. Many of my test families' kids were converted to salad lovers using this game!	4 and up
18. The Slow Food Experiment	page 161	The pace at which we eat our food influences how much we enjoy it. In general, the slower we eat, the better.	6 and up
19. The Same Food Three Ways Experiment	page 162	Food can taste dramatically different, depending on preparation style. That's why variety is fun.	4 and up
20. The Taste of Place Game	page 164	The concept of *terroir*, a French word that roughly translates as the "taste of place."	6 and up

Recipes for Raising an Adventurous Eater

These recipes are simple but tasty, with classic flavor combinations: carrot soup gets a dash of coriander, squash is paired with sage, green beans are matched up with almonds, and so on. These dishes are also quick to make: they take, on average, 10 minutes to prepare.

The recipes are designed to reinforce the idea of one family, one meal: every recipe is designed for adults to enjoy along with their kids. This means healthy eating for the whole family and less work for you—no more short-order cooking!

Most important, these recipes are designed to enable you to teach your child to like eating a range of fruits and vegetables. They follow a simple "laddering" approach, organized by age, that gradually introduces more complex tastes and textures as your child grows older. Three or four different recipes are provided for each specific fruit or vegetable, to correspond to the following different age groups:

(A) **babies** learning to eat solids (approximately 9 to 12 months)

(B) **older babies** comfortable chewing soft foods (12 to 36 months)

(C) **toddlers** (36 months to 5 years)

(D) **school-age kids** (6 years and up).

(Note: where a section does not include a recipe for babies it is because the main ingredient is not recommended for babies under 12 months.)

By the time your child is ready for school, they should be ready to eat like a grown-up! If you have older children, don't worry: you can start them on any rung of the ladder at any time. Even the baby recipes—many of which are simple soups—are designed to be eaten and enjoyed by kids and adults of all ages.

Introducing new foods to babies: The issue of allergies

The issue of when and how to introduce potentially allergenic foods is a matter of ongoing debate, and pediatric advice varies between countries. If you or someone in your family has a history of food allergies or asthma, consult your pediatrician before introducing your baby to solid foods and create a plan for adding new foods to your baby's diet. Allow an interval of time between introducing each new food so that you can monitor for a reaction. To play it safe, and as per United States FDA recommendations, the following recipes for babies do not use unpasteurized honey, raw eggs, processed meats, unpasteurized cheeses, peanuts, tree nuts (such as almonds, walnuts, and pecans), soybeans, wheat, or shellfish.

BROCCOLI

A GEORGE'S
BROCCOLI PUREE

B MOLLIE'S ENCHANTED
BROCCOLI RAINFOREST

C PARTY PASTA

D FRENCH MINESTRONE SOUP

George's Broccoli Purée

Special equipment: food processor or blender
Preparation: 5 minutes
Cooking: 6 minutes
Servings: 3 or 4 baby jars

Getting babies used to the taste and color of broccoli when they're still young is a great idea. It's one of the mildest green vegetables you can serve. In this recipe, it pairs well with other vegetables such as sweet potato or carrot. The thyme or tarragon (both optional) will bring out the flavor of both the carrot and broccoli, and the sweet potato adds richness. Don't be afraid to add the butter (or olive oil): it evens out the taste and makes this dish rich and satisfying. Even cautious babies will love this one!

60g peeled and chopped sweet potato
60g peeled and chopped carrot
45g small broccoli florets (no stems)
Pinch chopped fresh thyme or tarragon leaves, optional
Dab unsalted butter (or 1 teaspoon olive oil), optional
Pinch sea salt, optional

1. In a small saucepan over medium-low heat, bring 500ml of water to a boil. Add the sweet potato, then top with the carrot. Do not stir. Cover, increase heat to high, and cook for 3 minutes. Add the broccoli, reduce the heat to medium-high, and cook for 3 to 4 minutes, or until the vegetables are tender. Strain the vegetables, reserving the cooking liquid to make the purée.
2. Transfer the vegetables to a food processor (or use a blender) and purée, adding enough cooking liquid to

create a smooth consistency (start with 60ml, adding more as needed). To serve, top with a dab of butter (kids love watching it melt) and a small pinch of sea salt (if the butter in unsalted), if desired.

My kids thoroughly enjoyed the purée! It was easy to make. I kept it nice and chunky and added thyme. They took some bites, but after I added butter and sea salt, they inhaled it!

—Meg

Mollie's Enchanted Broccoli Rainforest

Special equipment: baking dish
Preparation: 5 minutes
Cooking: 20 minutes
Servings: 2 adults and 2 children (as a side dish)

This recipe is a little homage to Mollie Katzen, author of the *Enchanted Broccoli Rainforest*. It's one of my favorite kids' cookbooks because of the way it approaches vegetables—as something fun, interesting, and exciting!

I used this recipe to get my resistant younger daughter to start eating broccoli. She referred to them as "trees" for a while and would nibble daintily on the "leaves" (refusing to eat the "trunks"). Luckily this was a passing phase, helped by the fact that my husband likes broccoli stalks. After seeing him enjoy them for a while, she began eating each and every morsel.

1 head broccoli, cut into small florets
2 tablespoons olive oil
30g finely grated Parmesan cheese

30g dried breadcrumbs
Pinch chopped fresh thyme or tarragon, optional
Sea salt and ground black pepper, optional
1 tablespoon fresh lemon juice
2 tablespoons orange juice

1. Preheat the oven to 190°C/gas 5.
2. In a bowl, combine broccoli and oil and toss to coat. Transfer to a baking dish and add enough water to cover the bottom half of the broccoli. Roast in the oven for 20 minutes, or until the broccoli is tender. Drain the broccoli and set aside (see Notes).
3. In a bowl, combine the Parmesan, breadcrumbs, thyme, and salt and pepper, if using.
4. In a small bowl, combine the lemon and orange juices. Just before serving, pour the lemon-orange juice mixture over the broccoli and toss to coat. Add the breadcrumb mixture and toss to coat well.

Notes:
For younger babies (up until about 18 months), you'll probably want to set aside several broccoli florets before roasting and boil them until extremely tender, 5 to 7 minutes (roasting will also work, but it will take a lot longer than 20 minutes). For the youngest babies, you can also skip the juice and breadcrumb mixtures in Steps 3 and 4; however, once babies start eating it, they'll love it!

When my kids were younger, I often served this dish with mashed potatoes or Marvelous Mashed Cauliflower (page 231), making a little mountain of mash and inserting the broccoli like trees—artfully arranged, they do look like a little forest!

Party Pasta

Special equipment: none
Preparation: 5 minutes
Cooking: 15 minutes
Servings: 2 adults and 2 children

I often serve this delicious dish at informal dinner parties (hence the name). The anchovies add a salty flavor that really livens up the broccoli without a fishy flavor, and their oily tang is balanced by the fresh taste of lemon. Plus anchovies, like other small cold-water fish, are incredibly nutritious. Combining this with a kids' favorite—pasta—makes this a winner for most children.

This dish was one of the top five favorites among all my test families. It was a surprise to most of them, because the combination of broccoli and anchovy can be a little intimidating. Trust me, it's delicious. Here's the score from the kids at the Alphabet Academy, who taste tested many of the recipes in this book: 22 out of 25 tried it, 17 finished it all, and 15 asked for seconds. Believe me, it's *that* good!

225g dried penne or farfalle pasta
½ head broccoli, cut into bite-size pieces
Juice of ½ lemon (about 2 tablespoons)
3 tablespoons olive oil
3 to 5 anchovies (double if you really like anchovies; see Notes)
30g grated Parmesan (fresh is best, but I often used the pre-grated kind)
30g dried breadcrumbs, optional
Pinch crushed red pepper, optional (for the more adventurous eaters in the family!)

1. Bring a large pot of water to a boil over medium-high heat. Add the pasta and cook according to the package instructions, until al dente. Strain the pasta, reserving the cooking liquid for the sauce.
2. Meanwhile, bring a medium saucepan half-filled with water to a boil over medium-high heat. Add the broccoli and cook until just tender, 4 to 6 minutes. Drain the broccoli, transfer it to a bowl, and toss it with the lemon juice.
3. While the broccoli is cooking, in a large frying pan over medium-high heat, heat the oil. Add the anchovies and 60ml of the pasta cooking liquid. Sauté for 3 minutes, or until the anchovies soften and start to dissolve. Reduce the heat to low and cook until the liquid has reduced to a sauce, about 3 minutes.
4. Add the cooked pasta to the pan with the anchovy sauce and toss to coat. Add the prepared broccoli and toss to mix well. Serve topped with the Parmesan and breadcrumbs and crushed red pepper, if using.

Notes:

Anchovies are preserved in brine and then canned in oil (my preference) or salt water (too salty for my taste). If you do use anchovies packed in salt, rinse them well first.

If making this dish in advance, do not toss the lemon juice with the broccoli (it will turn brown over time). Instead, keep the broccoli and lemon juice separate, then just before serving toss them together and add to the pasta.

I was nervous about the anchovies: I've really never eaten them, and they just sounded gross to me. That's why I chose to make this dish. I feel like I need to let go of my own food hang-ups if I'm going to teach my kids to eat everything. And to my pleasant surprise, my three kids all ate this dish happily and without complaint!

—Stacy

French Minestrone Soup

Special equipment: none
Preparation: 20 minutes
Cooking: 20 minutes
Servings: 6 adults

This soup features *pistou* sauce, which is traditional in southern France where it is often served with pasta or spread on bread as well as used as a flavoring in soups and stews. There are many variations, but the basic principle is a sauce made from basil, garlic, and olive oil and often combined with Parmesan (much like pesto, but without the pine nuts). The rich flavor makes this veggie-packed soup worthy as a main dish.

Pistou can be used in so many dishes that I've included it as one of my Friendly Flavor Basics (see page 368). But my favorite is the Provençal *soupe au pistou*, a summer soup that includes vegetables like green beans, tomatoes, and zucchini.

In this minestrone recipe, the *pistou* is made with broccoli as well as basil, but without the garlic, making for a mild, tasty sauce that's somewhat creamier than the traditional version. The soup includes lots of yummy, healthy vegetables and even some pasta.

This soup travels well in thermoses (I send it in the kids' lunch bags), and the *pistou* freezes well (use ice-cube trays to make smaller servings you can easily thaw).

2 tablespoons olive oil
1 medium onion, diced, or 1 large leek, white part only, diced
2 carrots, peeled and diced
2 zucchini, diced
225g green beans, tips removed, cut into bite-size pieces
1 teaspoon dried thyme

130g frozen peas
100g small dried pasta (such as mini-macaroni or orecchiette)
100g chopped broccoli florets
400g can cannellini beans, drained (see Notes)
3 bay leaves
2.5 litres *Brodo* (page 364) or ready-to-use low-sodium vegetable stock
Pistou (page 368), for serving
2 tablespoons sun-dried tomato paste or puréed sun-dried tomatoes
1 teaspoon sea salt, optional (see Notes)

1. In a large soup pot, heat the oil over medium-low heat. Add the onion and cook, stirring occasionally, until translucent, 3 to 5 minutes. Add the carrots, zucchini, green beans, and thyme. Increase heat to medium-high and cook, stirring often, for 5 minutes, or until just tender (no longer, since the veggies will cook further in the soup). Add the peas, pasta, broccoli, beans, bay leaves, salt and *brodo*. Increase the heat to high and bring the soup to a boil, then reduce the heat to medium and simmer until the pasta is cooked, 6 to 8 minutes. Discard the bay leaves.
2. Ladle the soup into individual bowls. To each bowl, add about 1 teaspoon of *pistou* and a small spoonful of sun-dried tomato paste and stir gently (see Notes).

Notes:
To use dried beans in this recipe, place 200g of beans in a bowl, cover with water, and set aside overnight to soak. Drain and rinse the beans, then boil them in a saucepan of water over medium-high heat until tender, about 30 minutes. Drain and add to the soup.

The addition of *pistou* and sun-dried tomato paste is amazing in this dish! I often place bowls of *pistou* and sun-dried tomato paste on the table, as some people like to add more as they continue to eat. We also spread the *pistou* on bread, to accompany the soup—just as the French do.

Taste-Training Tip: *Pistou* can be used as a replacement for pesto with pasta.

> *My kids aren't big fans of soups in general, but this was a hit! After they each tried a little taste of the pistou, I put it on the center of the table and let them add it to the soup themselves. They all added it generously, and it seemed to make eating soup more fun for them!*
> —Roberta

CARROT

(A) TASTY ORANGE TRIO

(B) MAE WEST MASH

X-RAY VISION CARROTS!

(C) VICHY CARROTS

(D) GRATED CARROT SALAD

Tasty Orange Trio

Special equipment: steamer insert; food processor or blender
Preparation: 5 minutes
Cooking: 8 minutes
Servings: 6 to 8 baby jars

Carrots are a classic first food for babies, but they're often served plain. Not so in France! French parents introduce daily variations on familiar dishes to get their children used to new flavors, colors, and textures. Carrots, dill, and orange are a magical taste combination and often feature in adult soups. Parents can try this, too—you'll probably like it!

Once your baby is enjoying this purée, try substituting other herbs and spices for the dill, such as fresh parsley or coriander or ground cumin. This is a great base from which to introduce your baby to lots of variety early on, so be inventive!

250g peeled and chopped carrots
120ml orange juice
½ teaspoon dried dill

1. In a medium saucepan fitted with a steamer insert, bring 500ml water to a boil over high heat. Add the carrots, cover, and steam until tender, about 8 minutes. If you don't have a steamer, simmer the carrots in water over medium-high heat for about 5 minutes. Strain the carrots, reserving the cooking liquid.
2. In a food processor, combine the cooked carrots, orange juice, and dill and purée, slowly adding enough cooking liquid to reach the desired consistency. (Alternatively, you can use a blender to purée the carrots in the pan.)

Note:
This purée can easily be made the day before; the flavors intensify overnight. For adults or older kids, try adding more water to make a soup and season with a little grated ginger or cumin, plus salt, to taste.

Mae West Mash

Special equipment: none
Preparation: 5 minutes
Cooking: 15 minutes
Servings: 3 adults and 3 children

> *The only carrots that interest me are the number of carats in a diamond.*
> — Mae West

This recipe uses the classic French trio of carrots, celery (or celeriac), and onions (or leeks) known as *mirepoix*, which is used as the base for many French soups, stocks, and sauces. When served as a side dish (known as a *matignon*), the vegetables are gently sautéed in butter or olive oil over low heat, and herbs such as thyme are added. Set aside larger pieces of cooked vegetables as a perfect adult side dish for meat or lamb dishes, and gradually work your child up to an adult version of the mash they'll have come to love by leaving the purée more chunky as time goes on.

1 tablespoon olive oil or ½ tablespoon salted butter plus ½ tablespoon olive oil
1 small leek, diced, white part only, or diced onion
500g peeled and diced carrots
1 stalk celery, finely diced
120ml water, *Brodo* (page 364), or ready-to-use low-sodium vegetable stock

2 bay leaves
¼ teaspoon dried thyme
140g cubed cooked ham, optional

1. In a large frying pan over medium heat, heat the oil.
    Add the leek and sauté gently for about 3 minutes,
    until softened. Add the carrots and celery, increase
    the heat to medium-high, and cook for 3 minutes,
    stirring regularly. Add the water and bay leaves,
    increase the heat to high, and bring to a boil. Reduce
    the heat to medium, add the thyme, and simmer until
    the vegetables are tender and the liquid has evapo-
    rated, about 8 minutes. If using the ham, stir it in
    after 5 minutes. Remove the pan from the heat, dis-
    card the bay leaves, and serve—as is for older
    children and adults, or mashed for baby.

Vicious Carrots

Special equipment: large frying pan or wok
Preparation: 5 minutes
Cooking: 20 minutes
Servings: 2 adults and 3 children

While the proper name for this dish is "Vichy (*vee-shee*)
Carrots," my kids call these "Vicious Carrots." A visiting friend
once charmingly mispronounced the French name, and my
daughters couldn't stop laughing. What could be less vicious
than a carrot? Particularly in this seriously yummy recipe!
Needless to say, the name stuck. Legend has it this recipe is
adapted from a traditional French recipe that used Vichy
mineral water. It's a great side dish with chicken. Be sure to use
young, fresh carrots if you can find them—they'll be more
tender.

2 tablespoons salted butter
1 tablespoon liquid honey (see Note)
12 young, fresh carrots, peeled and sliced into bite-size coins
360ml *Brodo* (page 364) or ready-to-use low-sodium vegetable stock
1 tablespoon chopped fresh flat-leaf parsley leaves
Sea salt and ground black pepper, to taste

1. In a large frying pan or wok over medium heat, melt the butter. Add the honey and stir vigorously for 1 minute, or until the mixture starts to bubble slightly. Add the carrots and stir to coat them well.
2. Stir in the *brodo* (the carrots should be just covered). Bring the mixture to a boil, then reduce the heat to medium-high and simmer vigorously, uncovered, to allow the water to evaporate. (The dish should really be bubbling away!) Stir occasionally. After 15 to 20 minutes, the liquid will have reduced to a sauce (almost a glaze), and you'll have the most savory, melt-in-your-mouth carrots you've ever imagined eating. If it doesn't, pour off some of the liquid, turn up the heat slightly, and cook for a minute or two longer. Stir regularly (but gently) to make sure the carrots don't burn!
3. Sprinkle with parsley, salt, and pepper, and serve immediately. *Bon appétit!*

Note:
You can substitute an equal amount of sugar for the honey, if desired, but honey is better! Just remember that babies under 12 months aren't supposed to have unpasteurized honey.

Wow. The prep was so simple, and I can't say enough about the texture. You were right ... it took cooked carrots to an entirely different level.

—Lori

Grated Carrot Salad

Special equipment: box grater or food processor with shredding blade
Preparation: 10 minutes
Cooking: none
Servings: 2 adults and 3 children

Grated carrot salad is a favorite dish for French kids. They eat it regularly for school lunch, and it's popular at home as well. Even adults enjoy it as a starter.

The secret to this salad is in the texture: finely grated raw carrots that are simultaneously crisp and melt-in-your-mouth. The more finely grated the carrots, the more their natural sweetness comes out. For kids who have a hard time with crunchier textures, this might just be the dish that convinces them they love raw carrots. (You can also dress the salad with the Classic Vinaigrette on page 365.)

8 large carrots
30g finely chopped fresh flat-leaf parsley leaves (do not use dried parsley)
2 tablespoons extra virgin olive oil
Juice of 1 orange (about 120ml)
Juice of ½ lemon (about 2 tablespoons)
Pinch sea salt
½ teaspoon Dijon mustard, optional
Slices of lime, optional

1. Peel the carrots (important because the skin is often more bitter than the interior). Using a box grater or food processor fitted with the shredding blade, grate the carrots into fine shreds. (Food mills are popular

in France and make fine, delicate shredded carrot—
if you have one, use it!) Transfer the shredded carrots
to a large bowl. Add the parsley and mix to combine.

2. Make the dressing: In a small bowl, combine the oil,
orange and lemon juices, salt, and mustard, if using.
Taste and add more oil or lemon juice, as desired.

3. Mix just enough dressing into the carrots to coat
them lightly—do not overdress! Serve the salad at
room temperature or slightly chilled (see Notes),
topped with lime slices, if desired.

Notes:

This salad is tasty when prepared fresh, but will be even more
delicious if you let it marinate for a few hours, or even overnight,
in the refrigerator. The parsley taste will mellow, and the sweetness of the carrots will be more intense.

For another great flavor combination, substitute Coriander
Lime Dressing: Combine ⅛ teaspoon freshly grated lime zest,
2 tablespoons fresh lime juice, 2 tablespoons finely chopped fresh
coriander leaves, and 2 tablespoons extra virgin olive oil. It's a
fun way to introduce flavor variety after your children have
gotten used to the standard carrot salad recipe.

*I made the grated carrot salad with the coriander lime
dressing and the kids really enjoyed it. Will definitely
make it again. Nice and fresh, and simple to make!*
                                                    —Roberta

CAULIFLOWER

LOOKS JUST LIKE
MASHED POTATOES!

 A YUMMY YELLOW PURÉE

B MARVELOUS
MASHED CAULIFLOWER
(FAUX MASHED POTATOES)

 D JEWELED CAULIFLOWER RICE

 C CAULIFLOWER GRATIN

Yummy Yellow Purée

Special equipment: blender
Preparation: 5 minutes
Cooking: 8 minutes
Servings: 4 to 6 baby jars

The rich yellow color of this recipe comes from the turmeric, a spice widely used in Asia and particularly in Indian cooking. Turmeric is not spicy, but it still captures the warm, nutty essence of curry. It blends wonderfully with the cauliflower, giving it a subtle but interesting flavor.

Start by serving this dish to babies in small tasting portions: vegetables from the *Brassica* family (including cauliflower and broccoli) can give some people gassy tummies.

225g cauliflower florets
240ml *Brodo* (page 364) or ready-to-use vegetable stock
1 tablespoon salted butter
¼ teaspoon ground turmeric

1. Fill a medium saucepan with about 6 centimeters of water and bring to a boil over medium heat. Add the cauliflower and simmer for 7 to 8 minutes, or until the cauliflower is tender. Strain the cauliflower, reserving the cooking liquid.
2. In a blender, combine the cooked cauliflower, *brodo*, butter, and turmeric. Purée, adding enough cooking liquid to reach the desired consistency.

Note:
Turmeric stains bright yellow! Cover the carpets when you're serving this dish to baby.

Here's a fun idea: choose one bib to use solely for foods that stain (such as beets and curry)—you can call it the "curry bib"!

Taste-Training Tip: If you want some of the traditional spice of a curry in this dish, try substituting ½ teaspoon curry powder for the turmeric. My younger adventurous eater loved it, and even the older, more cautious one warmed up.

Marvelous Mashed Cauliflower (aka Faux Mashed Potatoes)

Special equipment: steamer insert or microwave-safe bowl; food processor
Preparation: 5 minutes
Cooking: 20 minutes stovetop/5 minutes microwave
Servings: 2 adults and 2 children

Mashed or creamed cauliflower is a healthy substitute for mashed potatoes: fewer calories, more nutrients! But that's not what I tell my kids. I simply say, "It's yummy." Magically, they seem to agree.

I find most mashed cauliflower recipes too watery, but this recipe is creamy—just like "real" mashed potatoes. Quite a few of my test families were dubious—but they all loved it!

1 head cauliflower, chopped into bite-size pieces
½ clove garlic, optional
2 tablespoons cream or milk (whatever you would normally use to make mashed potatoes)
2 tablespoons salted butter
Extra virgin olive oil, for garnish
Optional garnishes: 2 tablespoons chopped fresh coriander, parsley, chives, or dill or cooked bacon

1. In a medium saucepan fitted with a steamer, bring 500ml of water to a boil over high heat. Add the cauliflower and garlic, if using, and steam until very tender, 15 to 20 minutes. If you don't have a steamer, you can place the cauliflower and garlic in a microwave-safe bowl with 60ml water, cover, and microwave on high for 5 minutes.

2. Transfer the cooked cauliflower and garlic to a food processor and add the cream or milk and butter. Process until just smooth (if you over-process, it will get gooey). Serve hot, drizzled with olive oil and sprinkled with your garnish of choice.

My daughter couldn't believe this wasn't mashed potatoes! She votes it as a total success of a recipe.

—Jamie

Cauliflower Gratin

Special equipment: 20-cm baking dish
Preparation: 10 minutes
Cooking: 25 minutes
Servings: 2 adults and 2 children

I love this dish, in which cauliflower is baked in a classic French béchamel (white) sauce. It's deceptively delicious: who would have thought such a great casserole could be produced from such simple flavors? (This recipe appeared in *French Kids Eat Everything* and was such a hit with readers that I've included it here!)

1 head cauliflower, chopped into bite-size pieces
3 tablespoons salted butter

3 tablespoons plain flour
480ml milk
Sea salt and ground black pepper, to taste
Pinch nutmeg, optional

Topping:
30g dried breadcrumbs
30g grated Parmesan cheese

1. Preheat the oven to 180°C/gas 4 and butter a baking dish.
2. Bring a medium saucepan of water to a boil over medium-high heat. Add the cauliflower and cook it at a rolling boil for 7 to 8 minutes, or until it's tender but slightly crunchy. Drain and set aside.
3. Meanwhile, make the white sauce: In a large frying pan over medium heat, melt the butter. Sprinkle the flour into the butter and whisk until the flour is absorbed and forms a smooth paste. Immediately add the milk, whisking constantly (to avoid burning) until the sauce is the consistency of cream, about 3 minutes. (Don't overcook it; it will continue to thicken in the oven.) Stir in the salt and pepper, to taste, and the nutmeg, if using. Set aside.
4. In a small bowl, combine the breadcrumbs and Parmesan.
5. Place the cooked cauliflower in the prepared baking dish. Pour the white sauce evenly over the top, sprinkle with the breadcrumb mixture, and bake in the oven for 15 minutes, or until the top is golden brown and crunchy. Prepare to be converted to a cauliflower lover!

I made this last night with my 22-month-old; it came out quite pretty—and delicious! She had fun helping me layer the veggies and sprinkle the breadcrumbs on top, and she was so eager to eat it that she didn't want to wait for it to bake!

—*Alice*

Jeweled Cauliflower Rice

Special equipment: large frying pan or wok with a lid
Preparation: 15 minutes
Cooking: 20 minutes
Servings: 2 adults and 2 toddlers

This dish was inspired by a visit to one of my favorite Vancouver restaurants, Vij's, regularly voted one of the best Indian restaurants in North America. I had this dish only once, but I've been trying to recreate something like it ever since. This recipe has a few of my own twists (the addition of currants or raisins and the squeeze of fresh lime juice), and it isn't spicy like the adult version, but it will still please adult taste buds.

My kids love this dish, particularly the currants/raisins, which are soft, sweet, and slightly plump after being soaked in water. "They look like jewels," my younger daughter said once, and the name stuck. (Younger kids will have fun looking through their serving for their "jewels," but we have a rule: only one jewel per bite!)

1 teaspoon salted butter
280g basmati rice (see Notes)
2 tablespoons vegetable oil
1 teaspoon cumin seeds
1 medium onion, chopped
5 whole cloves
½ teaspoon ground turmeric
1 head cauliflower, chopped into bite-size pieces

70g currants or raisins, soaked in 120ml warm water
1 teaspoon sea salt, optional
15g finely chopped fresh flat-leaf parsley or coriander leaves
1 lime, for garnish

1. In a medium saucepan (with a lid) over medium-low heat, melt the butter. Add the rice, increase the heat to high, and cook, stirring vigorously, for 1 minute. Add 720ml of water and bring to a boil; as soon as the water is boiling, cover the pan and reduce the heat to low. Simmer until the water is absorbed, 12 to 15 minutes. Turn off the heat but keep the lid on, and let the rice rest for 2 minutes. Uncover and set aside.

2. Meanwhile, in a frying pan or wok over medium heat, heat the oil. Add the cumin seeds and let them sizzle in the pan for about 30 seconds, then add the onion and cloves. Sauté for 3 to 4 minutes, or until the onion is just starting to turn golden brown. Add the turmeric and sauté for 2 minutes, until the onion is well coated and the turmeric is absorbed. Add the cauliflower and currants with the soaking water, increase the heat to medium-high, and sauté for 5 minutes. Reduce the heat to medium-low, add salt, if using, cover, and cook for 5 minutes, or until the cauliflower is crisp-tender (cooked through but not too soft). Remove the cloves.

3. In a large bowl, combine the cooked rice, cauliflower mixture, and parsley and stir well. If desired, squeeze fresh lime juice over the top. Serve immediately (see Notes).

Notes:
The key to pilaf is that each grain of rice should be fluffy and separate. The rice shouldn't be sticky. To achieve this, either soak the rice in warm water for 20 minutes (and then discard the water) or, using a fine-mesh strainer, rinse the rice under running water,

rubbing it with your fingers to clean it. Either method will get rid of the starch that makes rice sticky.

Because rice can harbor bacteria that can cause food poisoning, this dish needs to be eaten immediately—no leftovers!

I made Jeweled Cauliflower Rice tonight. My 4-year-old was not too happy about it, saying it looked and smelled funny. Then she ate it and said, "It's delicious!" We couldn't get enough and even ran out.

—Babette

GREEN BEANS

GREEN
IS
GOOD!

(A) GREEN MACHINE PURÉE

(B) NIFTY NIÇOISE SOUP

(C) GREEN BEANS AMANDINE

(D) SALAD NIÇOISE

Green Machine Purée

Special equipment: steamer insert; blender or food
processor
Preparation: 5 minutes
Cooking: 8 minutes
Servings: makes about 360ml

Have you ever tasted store-bought baby "green bean purée"? It's
bland, stodgy, and extremely boring. That's too bad, because
green beans are actually quite tasty and packed full of nutrients.
If my first impression of a green bean was the jarred purée ...
well, *yuck!* This recipe introduces kids and babies to a great-tast-
ing version of a great-for-you food.

The garlic in this recipe is there for flavoring only (I often saw
French parents using garlic to subtly flavor their baby purées).
The secret is to cook the garlic with the other vegetables, but then
remove it before making your purée. It will add a nice bit of
flavor without the spicy bite.

I've suggested two methods below for cooking this dish: one
fast (boiling the veggies) and one slow (simmering/steaming them).
Slower cooking will retain more nutrients, but sometimes speed
is of the essence!

720ml water, *Brodo* (page 364), or ready-to-use low-sodium vegetable stock
100g chopped green beans
1 small zucchini, cut into large chunks
½ small clove garlic, optional
1 teaspoon dried basil or parsley

Fast method (boiling): Bring the water or *brodo* to a boil in a medium saucepan over medium-high heat. Add the beans, zucchini, and garlic, if using, and cook until the vegetables are tender, about 5 minutes. Reduce the heat to medium, add the basil, and simmer for 1 minute. Strain the vegetables, reserving the cooking liquid. Remove and discard the garlic. Return the vegetables to the pan with 240ml of the cooking liquid. Using a blender or food processor, purée the vegetables, adding enough cooking liquid to reach a desired consistency.

Slower method (steaming): In a medium saucepan fitted with a steamer insert, bring 480ml of water to a boil over high heat. Add the garlic direct to the boiling water. In the steamer, layer the beans, then the zucchini, and steam until the vegetables are tender, about 15 minutes. Remove and discard the garlic and reserve the cooking liquid. Transfer the vegetables to a blender or food processor and purée, slowly adding enough cooking liquid to reach the desired consistency.

Nifty Niçoise Soup

Special equipment: blender
Preparation: 5 minutes
Cooking: 15 minutes
Servings: 2 adults and 2 children (as small "starter soup")

This recipe uses the flavor pairing principle to create a mild dish that highlights the taste of green beans by pairing them with a hint of olives (an ingredient that brings out the flavor of the green beans). This 'anticipates' the ingredients of Salad Niçoise (a healthy, tasty French classic that both kids and adults will love). Don't be deceived by the small quantities of some of the ingredients: they add a hint of flavor without overpowering the soup. Less is more in this case! (Some of my taste-testing adults found this recipe bland, but some of their kids preferred it that way!)

This soup freezes well.

1 tablespoon olive oil
1 clove garlic, halved
2 carrots, peeled and cut into bite-size coins
100g green beans, trimmed and halved crosswise
720ml *Brodo* (page 364) or ready-to-use low-sodium vegetable stock
350g chopped zucchini
2 green or black olives, pitted (see Note)
½ teaspoon dried basil

Topping (optional for older kids and adults):
40g crumbled feta cheese
30g croutons

1. In a medium saucepan over medium heat, heat the oil for 1 minute. Add the garlic and sauté for 30 seconds, then add the carrots and green beans. Increase the heat to medium-high and simmer for 3 minutes, stirring occasionally. Add the *brodo,* zucchini, and olives. Increase the heat to high, bring to a boil, and boil for 1 minute. Reduce the heat to medium, add the basil, stirring to dissolve any clumps, and cook until the beans are soft, 5 to 8 minutes. Remove from the heat. Using a blender, purée the soup.

Note: Use high-quality black olives from a trusted source, as chemicals are sometimes used to artificially turn olives black.

Taste-Training Tip: If your children don't like olives, have them try even a tiny nibble of an olive beforehand. This will prepare them for the slight taste of olives in this soup.

I had the girls feel the olives beforehand. No one in my house (except me, of course) cares for green olives. I didn't tell them I was putting them in the soup, I just had them smell and feel them. They were certain: green olives look bad, smell bad, and surely taste bad. So when I poured the soup into the bowls, I was sure they wouldn't like it—but they did! No one could guess the aftertaste. I loved the looks on their faces when I told them it was green olives!

—Lori

Green Beans Amandine

Special equipment: none
Preparation: 5 minutes
Cooking: 15 minutes
Servings: 2 adults and 2 children (at least!)

This French dish is a much-loved American classic. My version of the recipe lightens it up a bit (less fat, more crunch), but the essential flavors are still there. This is a great way to enliven an old favorite—and a perfect match for that Sunday roast!

1 tablespoon salted butter
1 tablespoon olive oil
70g sliced almonds
675g fresh green beans, tips removed, chopped into bite-size pieces
Zest of ½ lemon
Sea salt and ground black pepper

1. Bring a large saucepan of water to a boil over high heat.

2. Meanwhile, in a large frying pan over medium heat, melt the butter in the oil. Add the almonds and sauté for 3 to 4 minutes, stirring often, until the almonds start to smell like they're toasting. (Pay attention— they can burn quickly!) Remove the frying pan from the heat and set aside.

3. When the water is boiling, add the green beans and reduce the heat to medium. Simmer the beans for 5 minutes, or until just tender. (Don't overcook or they'll be mushy!) Drain the beans, discarding the water.

4. Add the cooked beans to the pan with the almonds and increase the heat to medium-high. Cook, stirring continuously, for about 1 minute, then add the lemon zest and salt and pepper, to taste. Cook, stirring, for another 1 or 2 minutes to allow the flavors to mingle. (Optional: grate a little zest on top for added texture and color.) Serve immediately.

I gave Tobias (3) his own wedge of lemon to squeeze over the top, which made it more fun for him. He said "Oooh, crunchy!" about the almonds, so those were a hit.

—Martha

Salad Niçoise

Special equipment: none
Preparation: 20 minutes
Cooking: 12 minutes
Servings: 2 adults and 2 children

I started making this dish because my younger daughter (who loves everything from olives to stinky Roquefort cheese) went through an inconvenient phase where she didn't like eggs. Her older sister would eat them scrambled, hard-boiled, poached— you name it—but Claire had developed a bit of a mental block about them. So I made this salad with her, and she would pick out the things she liked. Gradually, ever so slowly, she'd begin trying bits of egg. Eventually she devoured them!

Traditionally, this classic French salad does not contain any cooked vegetables. It features raw vegetables, hard-boiled eggs, anchovies, olive oil, and, of course, niçoise olives! Lettuce, rice, and potatoes—ingredients made popular by Julia Child—aren't normally featured. Try it this way or add in your favorite ingredients—there are as many ways to make *salad niçoise* as there are chefs!

2 large eggs
200g green beans, trimmed and halved crosswise
½ head green lettuce (preferably romaine), torn into bite-size pieces
2 large ripe tomatoes, quartered
70g black niçoise olives, pitted
8 anchovy fillets, drained (if you buy them packed in oil) or 1 can tuna, drained

Dressing:
120ml extra virgin olive oil
60ml red wine vinegar
15g chopped fresh herbs (parsley and basil are best, but you can also use coriander)
Sea salt and ground black pepper, to taste
½ clove garlic, minced, optional

1. Put the eggs in a small saucepan and cover with 2.5 to 5 centimeters of cold water. Cover and bring the water to a boil over high heat. Once boiling, turn off the heat but leave the pan on the burner for 12 minutes—set your timer! (Cooking eggs this way keeps

the shells from cracking, keeps the egg whites tender, and avoids that green-grey rim around the yolks.) Rinse the eggs under cold running water, then peel them and set aside.

2. Meanwhile, bring a medium saucepan of water to a rolling boil over high heat. Add the green beans, reduce the heat to medium-high, and cook for 7 to 8 minutes, or until just tender. Drain the beans and set aside.

3. Quarter the eggs or chop into small pieces.

4. Place the lettuce in the bottom of a large, preferably shallow, serving bowl. Arrange the tomatoes, cooked eggs, cooked beans, olives, and anchovies over the top.

5. In a small bowl, whisk together the oil, vinegar, herbs, salt, pepper, and garlic, if using. Pour over the salad and serve immediately.

Taste-Training Tip: This is one of those dishes for which "combine your own" strategies sometimes work. On individual plates, lay out the lettuce together with the veggies that you know your child likes. Put the other ingredients in bowls on the table. Invite your child to add extra ingredients to make their own salad. Be sure you set the example of helping yourself to each bowl and enjoying the salad, too!

PEAS

A MINTY GREEN PUREE

Spinach +
Peas! Yum!

B EAT 'YER GREENS SOUP

C EASY NO-STIR PEA RISOTTO

D CHICKEN AND PEA CURRY

Minty Pea Purée

Special equipment: food processor or blender
Preparation: 2 minutes
Cooking: 8 minutes
Servings: about 480ml or 4 to 6 baby jars

This pea purée uses just a small amount of mint to gently introduce the taste, and adds zucchini to lighten the texture of the
purée, which makes it smooth and creamy. For an extra-creamy
taste, you can add yogurt, sour cream, milk, or any dairy substitute.

280g frozen peas, thawed
2 medium potatoes, peeled and chopped
3 to 4 fresh mint leaves
1 medium zucchini, peeled and sliced
2 tablespoons Greek yogurt, sour cream, or milk, optional
1 tbsp salted butter
Pinch sea salt

1. Bring 1 litre of water to a rolling boil in a medium
   saucepan over high heat. Add the peas, potato, and
   mint and return to a boil. Reduce the heat to
   medium-high and simmer for 5 minutes. Add the zucchini and cook for 3 minutes, until the potatoes are
   cooked through. Strain the vegetables, reserving the
   cooking liquid.
2. In the same pan, combine the cooked vegetables with
   240ml of the cooking liquid. Using a food processor
   or blender, purée until smooth. For a creamier purée,
   mix in the yogurt, if using. Stir in the butter and salt.
   If needed, add more cooking liquid to reach the desired

consistency. For a very fine purée, push the mixture through a fine-mesh sieve before serving. Serve warm.

Taste-Testing Tip: This is a great recipe to use if you would like to introduce the taste of fish to babies (some pediatricians recommend introducing fish at 9 months, others at 12 months). Simply add 60g of fresh white fish (such as sole) when you cook the peas, first making sure there are no fish bones, and purée as directed. *Voilà!*

Eat Yer Greens Soup with Fresh Mint Cream

Special equipment: blender or food processor
Preparation: 5 minutes
Cooking: 20 minutes
Servings: 2 adults and 2 children

Peas are rich in minerals, vitamins, and fiber, and they taste good—slightly sweet and quite flavorful. If you introduce them to kids early, most will learn to love them. Plus, peas are a great base from which to springboard to more adventurous taste training. Once your child has learned to love peas, you can start adding other tastes. This recipe combines the flavors of the Minty Pea Purée (opposite) and Spinach Purée (page 262) for a lovely soup that the whole family can eat together.

This soup freezes well, but make the Fresh Mint Cream just before serving.

3 tablespoons salted butter
1 medium onion, chopped
½ teaspoon mild curry powder (see Notes)
285g frozen peas, thawed

285g frozen chopped spinach, thawed
720ml *Brodo* (page 364) or ready-to-use vegetable or chicken
stock
4 tablespoons chopped fresh mint leaves
½ teaspoon sea salt, optional
½ teaspoon ground black pepper
240ml milk (see Notes)

Fresh Mint Cream:
2 tablespoons chopped fresh mint leaves
120ml crème fraîche

1. In a large saucepan over medium heat, melt the butter. Add the onion and curry powder, stirring well, and sauté until the onion starts to turn golden, 4 or 5 minutes.
2. Add the peas, spinach, and *brodo*. Bring the mixture to a boil, then reduce the heat to medium-low and simmer for 5 minutes. Add the mint and simmer for 5 minutes, or until the peas are tender.
3. Meanwhile, make the Fresh Mint Cream: In a blender, combine the mint and crème fraîche and purée until smooth. Set aside.
4. Remove the soup from the heat and stir in the milk and salt and pepper, if using. Transfer the mixture to a blender or food processor and purée until completely smooth. Serve immediately, topped with the mint cream. (I sometimes make little happy faces for the kids—one drop for each eye, a dollop for the nose, a curly swirl for the mouth—but they love to make up their own designs, too!)

Notes:
For more tentative kids, omit the curry powder. As their tastes change, you can introduce it, increasing the amount of curry powder to 1 teaspoon or more.

If needed, you can use a milk substitute; it will, however, change the texture considerably.

Easy No-Stir Pea Risotto

Special equipment: none
Preparation: 5 minutes
Cooking: 30 minutes
Servings: 2 adults and 3 children (as a main course with generous servings)

This dish was one of the top five favorites among all my test families. The kids at the Alphabet Academy gave it an enthusiastic thumbs up: 15 out of 17 preschoolers loved it and wanted more!

It's funny, because this dish almost didn't make it into the book. Given my absentmindedness—my husband christened me *"La Reine des Casseroles Brûlés"* (Queen of Burned Pots) soon after we were married—I was terrified of making risotto until an Italian friend of mine showed me this oven-baked version that doesn't require you to stir, and stir, and stir—magic! The texture is a bit different than the stovetop version—a tiny bit less creamy—but it's still delicious.

1.25 litres *Brodo* (page 364) or ready-to-use low-sodium vegetable or chicken stock
290g risotto rice (see Notes)
100g grated Parmesan cheese
3 tablespoons salted butter
½ teaspoon sea salt, optional (see Notes)
1 teaspoon ground black pepper
130g frozen peas, thawed
1 teaspoon fresh lemon juice, optional

1. Preheat the oven to 180°C/gas 4. In a medium saucepan over medium-low heat, bring the *brodo* to a simmer.
2. In a large baking dish, combine the rice and 1 litre of the hot stock. Cover (use foil, if necessary) and bake in the oven for 30 minutes, until most of the liquid is absorbed and the rice is just slightly firm to the bite (al dente).
3. Remove the dish from the oven and stir in the Parmesan, remaining 240ml of hot stock, butter, salt, if using, and pepper. Stir vigorously until the rice is thick and creamy, 2 to 3 minutes. Add the peas and stir until heated through. Add the lemon juice, if using. Serve immediately (it tends to get thicker and stodgier if you wait).

Notes:
I prefer to use Carnaroli or Arborio rice for this dish. Some readers have reported success using brown rice—if that is all you have, give it a go!

Parmesan cheese is salty, so I would not add too much salt to this dish—salt it at the table if necessary.

Because rice can harbor bacteria that can cause food poisoning, this dish needs to be eaten immediately and not used for leftovers. Plus, the texture will get mushy.

I just can't get enough of this recipe. It's too easy for such buttery-risotto results! The girls were lukewarm about it on the first try, and on the second attempt—in which it was essentially the same—they cleaned their bowls and asked why hadn't I made this before. "So delicious!" Kids are funny.

—*Lori*

Chicken and Pea Curry

Special equipment: wok or large deep frying pan
Preparation: 10 minutes
Cooking: 20 minutes
Servings: 2 adults and 2 children (as a main course)

Thanks to the Easy No-Stir Pea Risotto (page 249) and Eat Yer Greens Soup (page 247) recipes, your child is now familiar with the texture of peas and rice, as well as the taste of turmeric—a key ingredient in curry. Time for the big league! This very mild curry is a great way to introduce your child to the taste of Indian food. I serve this curry with rice and mango chutney. *Yum!*

In my family we experiment with this recipe: sometimes I'll add thinly sliced carrot, or a garlic clove; other times I leave out the sweet potato. The possibilities are endless! But do make sure to try this recipe with the apple—the sweetness offsets the curry, and the melt-in-your-mouth texture of the cooked apple is a nice complement to the chicken.

1 tablespoon vegetable oil
1 tablespoon mild curry paste (see Notes)
1 tablespoon tomato purée
1 medium sweet potato, peeled and cut into bite-size pieces
1 carrot, peeled and diced
1 large apple, peeled, cored, and thinly sliced
2 large boneless skinless chicken breasts, cut into bite-size pieces
400g can coconut milk
240ml *Brodo* (page 364) or ready-to-use low-sodium vegetable or chicken stock
285g bag frozen peas (or equivalent fresh)
Chopped fresh coriander, for garnish
Cooked rice, for serving

Mango chutney, for serving

1. In a wok or frying pan over high heat, heat the oil. Stir in the curry paste and gently cook for 1 minute. Add the tomato purée, sweet potato, carrot, apple, and chicken, stirring until well coated. Cook, stirring often, for 5 minutes. Pour in the coconut milk and *brodo*. Increase the heat to high and bring to a boil. Once boiling, immediately reduce the heat to medium and simmer for 5 minutes. Add the peas and simmer for 5 minutes more, until tender (but not mushy). Serve over cooked rice with mango chutney on the side. *Delish!*

Notes:

I like to use Korma curry paste in this recipe. Adventurous eaters may want to increase the amount used to 2 tablespoons!

If you feel this dish needs salt, just sprinkle a tiny pinch of salt on each dish before serving. You'll taste the salt more, but actually be eating less.

The spice level was perfect for the kids, and they really enjoyed it. My boys' comments: my 7-year-old said, "Good! But maybe add some cashews to it the next time" (I kid you not); my 5-year-old said, "I like that it's kind of sugary" (he's referring to the sweetness of the apples); and my 3-year-old said, "I like the peas and the chicken." I thought it was great and will definitely make it again.

—Roberta

PEPPERS

HOW DEEP
CAN YOU DIP IN?

A ROASTED RED PEPPER
AND TOMATO SOUP

B RED ROCKET HUMMUS

C PINWHEEL PEPPER WRAPS

D RATATOUILLE
(SOUTHERN FRENCH STEW)

Roasted Red Pepper and Tomato Soup

Special equipment: blender
Preparation: 5 minutes
Cooking: 15 minutes
Servings: 2 adults and 2 children

This recipe features roasted and peeled peppers but let me reassure you: I have tried this recipe with both store-bought and fresh, do-it-yourself roasted red peppers, and the soup made with the store-bought kind is just as good. (Of course, if you want to roast them yourself, be my guest!)

Some adult versions of this recipe use sugar and chicken stock but I prefer to use the juice of one orange and vegetable stock—the soup is naturally sweet, and the tomato and pepper flavors are complemented, but not overpowered, by the stock.

This soup freezes well.

1 tablespoon olive oil
¼ onion, chopped
½ small garlic clove (see Note)
5 large ripe tomatoes, cored and quartered
2 large or 3 small roasted red peppers
2 tablespoons chopped fresh basil leaves
1 litre *Brodo* (page 364) or ready-to-use low-sodium vegetable stock
Juice of 1 orange (about 120ml)
Parmesan cheese, thinly sliced, optional
Fresh basil leaves, for garnish, optional

1. In a large saucepan over medium heat, heat the oil. Add the onion and garlic and sauté until the onion is translucent, about 3 minutes. Increase the heat to

high and add the tomatoes, red peppers, and basil. Cook, stirring continuously, for 1 minute. Stir in the *brodo* then reduce the heat to medium and simmer for 10 minutes. Stir in the orange juice.

2. Using a blender, purée the soup until creamy smooth. Serve immediately, topped with Parmesan and a basil leaf, if desired (the cheese will melt into the soup, making it more creamy).

Note: I don't chop the garlic because small pieces can burn. The garlic will get puréed at the end anyway.

Adult Serving Tip: This soup is delicious, hot or cold, garnished with croutons. Stirring a bit of basil or coriander pesto into this soup makes it divine! Also try serving this with a black olive tapenade on the side.

> *This soup was great. Kids loved it, husband loved it. I put crackers on the side. I didn't get many comments; that's what I noticed happens when they like it—they just eat it up!*
>
> —Françoise

Red Rocket Hummus

Special equipment: steamer insert; food processor
Preparation: 10 minutes
Cooking: 10 minutes
Servings: 2 adults and 2 children or about 12 baby jars

This recipe uses cream. It offsets the acidity of the peppers and tomatoes while enhancing their flavor (the French are never afraid of using a little fat). If you prefer, you can substitute yogurt.

For older babies, you can add 1 stalk of fennel, a bay leaf, and ½ clove of garlic to gently flavor it (but make sure you remove them before you purée it!).

Like most of the purée recipes in this book, this makes a lovely dish for adults—it's really a red pepper hummus in disguise!

This hummus freezes well.

½ clove garlic, optional (see Notes)
1 ripe tomato, quartered
1 red pepper, cored, seeded, and sliced
400g can chickpeas, rinsed and drained
1 tablespoon whipping cream (see Notes)
1 tablespoon extra virgin olive oil
Juice of ½ lemon (about 2 tablespoons)
Pinch sea salt, optional

1. In a medium saucepan fitted with a steamer insert, bring 720ml of water to a boil over medium heat. Add the garlic, if using, directly to the water. In the steamer, cook the tomato and red pepper for 7 to 8 minutes, or until the red pepper is tender. Strain the tomato and pepper, reserving the cooking liquid and discarding the garlic.

2. In a food processor, combine the cooked tomato and red pepper with the chickpeas, cream, oil, and lemon juice and purée until smooth. If too thick, slowly add enough cooking liquid to reach the desired consistency. (Adults may want to add the salt to their serving.)

Notes:
As your child grows, you can increase the intensity of the garlic in the recipe. For younger babies, boil the garlic in the water while you're steaming the tomato and pepper, then discard the garlic, as described in the recipe; the hummus will have just a hint

of garlic flavor. For older kids, rather than discarding the cooked garlic, add it to the purée. This will lend a nice flavor to the hummus and is a lovely introduction to garlic!

If desired, you can substitute an equal amount of full-fat yogurt for the cream. For babies over 12 months, try substituting 1 tablespoon light tahini.

Pinwheel Pepper Wraps

Special equipment: none
Preparation: 5 minutes
Cooking: none
Servings: 2 adults and 2 children

This simple recipe combines the crunchy texture of fresh red pepper with a smooth, savory cream cheese filling. These are great for school lunches. They're also a good recipe on which to test out your marketing tactics. The color swirls look fun; ask kids to come up with interesting names!

It really helps to warm the tortillas first: warm, fresh tortillas bring out the flavors of the other ingredients, and they are much easier to chew.

4 small flour tortillas
4 tablespoons cream cheese or Red Rocket Hummus (page 255)
1 red pepper, cored, seeded, and finely chopped

Optional fillings (as your child grows older):
Avocado slices
Cooked sliced chicken
Roasted red pepper spread
Chopped fresh basil leaves

1. In a dry frying pan over medium-low heat, gently warm the tortillas on each side. Transfer the tortillas to a clean work surface and spread 1 tablespoon of the cream cheese on top of each tortilla, then sprinkle each evenly with 1 tablespoon red pepper. Fold the sides and bottom of each tortilla up over the filling, then roll tightly to close. Using a sharp knife, slice the rolls diagonally into 1.5cm-thick slices and serve immediately.

Note: Some smaller children may have trouble chewing these. You can cut the pinwheels into little pieces so they can eat them with a fork (or fingers!).

The children in our classrooms were very eager to see what was going to be served today! The votes are in: out of 40, 34 would like to have it on our menu. We recorded a lot of "crunchy," "sweet," "yummy, I want more!" and "great mix of crunchy and chewy!" We also heard, "I've never liked peppers, but now I like them—they are so delicious." Our favorite: "Mmmm, I tasted it with my taste bugs!"

—*Alphabet Academy*

Ratatouille (Southern French Stew)

Special equipment: none
Preparation: 10 minutes
Cooking: 25 minutes
Servings: 2 adults and 2 children (as a main dish)

Ratatouille (*ra-ta-too-ee*) is traditionally a summer dish (these vegetables all ripen in late summer), but it's one of my children's favorite dishes at any time of the year.

There are many ways to make ratatouille, but they basically divide into two approaches. The "slow food" approach insists that each vegetable needs to be peeled, then sautéed individually, and then the entire dish slowly roasted for hours. I've had it made this way—and it is indeed totally delicious—but it's also unrealistically time-consuming. The "grandmother's stew" approach (my preference) insists that this was always a simple dish that was left to simmer on the stove for hours, with no fuss. This is the way I make it, as a more liquid dish with a yummy stock that kids love. You don't need to peel the veggies (but you may if you like).

We also use ratatouille as a pasta sauce (you might want to simmer it for a bit longer, to thicken it up a bit more), eat it with roast chicken, and even use it as an ingredient in quiche. Or you can add chicken stock and blend it as a soup (remove the bay leaves first!), which freezes really well.

3 tablespoons olive oil
2 large leeks, white and green parts, finely sliced
2 teaspoons sea salt
1 medium eggplant, peeled and cut into 2.5-cm chunks
1 clove garlic, halved
8 to 10 large ripe tomatoes, cored and quartered
1 red pepper, cored, seeded, and cut into big chunks
1 large zucchini, peeled and cut into 1.5-cm chunks
1 tablespoon herbes de Provence (usually includes rosemary, thyme, basil, marjoram)
2 bay leaves
1 generous tablespoon liquid honey or dark brown sugar or pure maple syrup
½ teaspoon ground black pepper
30g finely chopped fresh flat-leaf parsley leaves

1. In a large saucepan over medium-low heat, heat the oil. Add the leek and ½ teaspoon salt and sauté for about 5 minutes, or until the leeks are just starting to turn golden. Add the eggplant and garlic and stir well; cover and sauté for another 5 minutes, or until the eggplant is tender. Add the tomatoes, red pepper, zucchini, herbs, bay leaves, honey, remaining salt, pepper, and parsley. Cover, increase the heat to high, bring to a near-boil, then reduce the heat to medium, and cook, stirring occasionally, until all of the vegetables are perfectly tender, 10 to 15 minutes. Discard the bay leaves. Serve warm.

Time-saving Tip: This dish comes together quickly because it cooks in stages: while one veggie is sautéing, you can chop the next one.

Note: This dish tastes great when first cooked, but is even better after it has sat for a few hours, which allows the flavors to meld. I try to make it the night before, cool it, and refrigerate it overnight. When reheated, the flavors become more savory. The restaurant La Note in Berkeley, California, serves ratatouille on a bed of couscous, topped with poached eggs; this transforms it from a side dish into a main course.

SPINACH

B SOPHIE'S SPINACH SURPRISE

C SPEEDY SALMON SPINACH LASAGNA

MAKE A FUNNY FACE!

D WARM SPINACH CITRUS SALAD

Sophie's Spinach Surprise

Special equipment: blender
Preparation: 2 minutes
Cooking: 5 minutes
Servings: about 4 baby jars

This recipe appeared in *French Kids Eat Everything*, as it was one of the first dishes I made to encourage our daughters to eat more vegetables. It worked like a charm! Several years later—even though they both eventually graduated to other green vegetables—my kids still love this dish (which I now serve as a starter soup in small ramekins).

This dish is mild and incredibly smooth and is an easy way to introduce your children to green vegetables. The zucchini provides a light, almost fluffy, melt-in-your-mouth texture, so that the spinach tastes airy and almost sweet. If you think the dish is still bitter (although I never do), add a tiny bit of honey before serving (or use a little less spinach).

This dish freezes wonderfully well and reheats quickly. But you may want to add a little water when reheating, as it tends to thicken slightly after being frozen.

1 medium or large zucchini, peeled and chopped
2 or 3 big handfuls baby spinach leaves
1 teaspoon salted butter, optional
Whipping cream, optional
Pinch sea salt, optional

1. In a medium saucepan over high heat, combine the zucchini and 240ml of water. Bring to a boil, reduce the heat to medium, and simmer until the zucchini becomes transparent, about 2 minutes. Stir in the

spinach and cook for 1 or 2 minutes, just until the spinach wilts. (Don't overcook the spinach or it will become slimy!) Strain the vegetables, reserving the cooking liquid. Remove the pan from the heat and, using a blender, purée until perfectly smooth, adding enough cooking liquid to reach a desired consistency. Stir in butter, cream, and salt, if desired.

Taste-Training Tips:
I've served spinach to both of my children for years, without any issues—spinach is one of their favorite foods!—however, because of its potentially high nitrate content, you should avoid serving spinach to babies younger than 12 months old and limit the amount you serve at any one sitting. Serve the purée in a small bowl as a side dish rather than the main meal (I find that a little goes a long way.) Top it with tiny dabs of butter in the form of a happy face—your child will love to watch them melt. Encourage your child to "catch" the eyes (or nose or mouth) before they disappear!

Older kids and adults will enjoy this with the optional cream, butter, and salt, but little ones will eat this plain and love it, so serve it to them plain first!

Speedy Salmon Spinach Lasagna

Special equipment: 32- x 22-cm baking dish
Preparation: 20 minutes
Cooking: 40 minutes
Servings: 4 adults and 2 children, with generous servings

This is a recipe the whole family will enjoy, and it's one of the dishes I love serving to guests, particularly out-of-town visitors, for whom I'll use fresh salmon (one of Vancouver's local delicacies) when it's in season. The salmon becomes very tender as it bakes in the béchamel sauce and is offset by the smooth firmness of the ricotta-spinach layers. Both of my toddlers liked this lasagna.

This recipe works just as well with canned salmon (in fact, some members of my family think it's even better). In recognition that good, fresh ingredients are sometimes hard to find, I've included frozen and canned options for this recipe—that's what makes it speedy!

3 tablespoons salted butter
3 tablespoons plain flour
720ml milk
170–200g can wild salmon (remove skin and any large bones)
1 tablespoon dried oregano
1 teaspoon sea salt, optional
1 teaspoon ground black pepper, optional
450g ricotta cheese
285g thawed and drained frozen spinach or 1 small bunch fresh spinach, cut into 1.5-cm pieces
2 large eggs
1 teaspoon ground cinnamon
12 to 16 fresh or cooked lasagna sheets (see Note)
230g shredded Cheddar cheese
60g grated Parmesan cheese
1 to 2 tablespoons chopped capers, for garnish, optional

1. Preheat the oven to 190°C/gas 5.
2. Make the salmon in béchamel sauce: In a medium saucepan over high heat, melt the butter. Add the flour and cook, whisking constantly, for 1 minute, until a smooth paste forms. Whisk in the milk and cook for 1 minute, or until the paste dissolves. Reduce the heat to medium and cook, stirring constantly, until the sauce begins to thicken, 3 to 4 minutes. Add the salmon, stirring well to break up the chunks, and the oregano and salt and pepper, if using. Set aside.

3. In a large bowl, stir together the ricotta, spinach, eggs, and cinnamon.

4. In a baking dish, assemble the lasagna by layering the ingredients in the following order (as you make the layers, be sure the lasagna sheets are in contact with the béchamel sauce everywhere—if they don't absorb the sauce, they'll stay hard):

   • Half the salmon béchamel sauce
   • 1 layer lasagna sheets
   • All the spinach-ricotta filling
   • 1 layer lasagna sheets
   • All but about 60ml remaining salmon béchamel sauce (reserve some for the top)
   • 1 layer lasagna sheets

5. Drizzle the top of the lasagna with the reserved salmon béchamel. Sprinkle evenly with the Cheddar, Parmesan, and, if using, capers (the capers add a bit of zing for older kids and adults). Bake in the oven for 30 minutes, or until the topping is golden and crunchy and the filling is bubbling. Set aside to cool for at least 10 minutes before serving (the filling is piping hot and, cooled slightly, the lasagna will be much firmer and hold its shape better when sliced, as the ricotta filling helps the pieces hold their shape).

Note: You'll need enough lasagna sheets to create 3 layers, using 3 to 4 sheets per layer.

Serving Tip: This is a mild, almost delicate lasagna. Try serving it after a fresh starter salad with a tangy vinaigrette; the tastes will complement one another nicely. For a nice garnish, sprinkle a bit of dried oregano or parsley on top.

*To be honest, I was worried about this one. It sounded
like an odd combo, and my kids are used to more traditional lasagna. My first pleasant surprise was the canned
salmon. I have never used it before. It was great and not
at all fishy! The lasagna was really interesting. It looked
beautiful and cut nicely. My 7-year-old (my pickiest eater)
did the best with it. On a scale of 1 to 10, he gave it a
"150."*

—Stacy

Warm Spinach Citrus Salad

Special equipment: none
Preparation: 5 minutes
Cooking: 2 minutes
Servings: 2 adults and 2 children (small servings)

My kids now love lettuce and spinach. But I admit that it took
a while. We started off with a toddler version of this salad, in
which I served the ingredients as a happy face on a plate (5 or 6
spinach leaves for hair, mandarin orange pieces for eyes, half a
cherry tomato for a nose, and so on). These happy faces take
only a minute to make (as you pluck the pieces out of the salad
you've made for the adults), and the kids can even help make
them when they are older. The kids would dip their pieces in
homemade vinaigrette, getting used to the taste and texture of
salad, which we served first, before the main course. Eventually
they proudly graduated to "grown-up" salad (although I admit
to still surprising my younger one, now in kindergarten, with a
salad happy face once in a while!).

If you're starting with toddlers, remember that the happy
face version isn't necessarily about your children eating a lot
of salad. It's about them learning to *like the idea* of eating

salad. Most kids won't start eating larger quantities until they're older.

225g loosely packed baby spinach (see Note)
2 mandarin oranges or clementines, peeled and separated into segments
75g cherry tomatoes, halved
60ml Classic Vinaigrette (page 365)

1. Heat a medium saucepan over medium heat. Wash the spinach under cool running water, then immediately place it in the pan and toss as you would a salad. As soon as you hear a hissing sound (which means that the water is evaporating off of the spinach), remove the pan from the heat. The spinach should be slightly (*just* slightly!) wilted.

2. In a medium bowl, combine most of the oranges and tomatoes. Add the cooked spinach, then top with the remaining oranges and tomatoes. Don't toss the salad or the spinach will lose volume. Serve immediately with the vinaigrette on the side. (You can serve the vinaigrette mixed in as well, but be sure not to over-toss the salad.)

Note: Baby spinach leaves are smaller and quite tender compared with regular spinach leaves. They are wonderful combined with the slightly acidic oranges and tomatoes, and the vitamin C in the citrus and tomatoes helps you absorb the iron in the spinach!

I decided to make the salad, as my kids have a phobia about salads! I realized that making the happy face is still worth it for 6- and 9-year-olds—they loved it! And warming up the spinach made all the difference; they liked the soft texture.

—Françoise

SQUASH

SQUASH ME, PLEASE!

A SQUISH SQUASH SOUP

B ROAST SQUASH WITH MAPLE DRESSING

C SQUASH SAGE SOUP

D MILD THAI SQUASH CURRY

Squish Squash

Special equipment: blender or food processor
Preparation: 5 minutes
Cooking: 50 minutes
Servings: 480 to 720ml (depending how big your squash is)

This purée takes a little longer to prepare than most of the other recipes in the book, but it has two great advantages: it makes a delicious adult side dish (I've provided quantities based on the assumption that adults will eat it, too) and the recipe's funny name might convince reluctant eaters to try a bite or two!

1 large butternut squash
1 tablespoon salted butter or vegetable oil
2 ripe pears or apples, peeled, cored, and quartered
Pinch sea salt, optional
½ teaspoon ground cinnamon, optional
Zest of ½ orange, optional

1. Preheat the oven to 200°C/gas 6.
2. Halve the squash lengthwise and remove the seeds and strings. Rub the insides with butter. Place squash, cut-side down, in a baking dish with 60ml of water. Bake in the oven for 30 minutes, then add the pears. Bake for another 15 to 20 minutes, or until the squash is tender when pricked with a fork.
3. Remove the dish from oven and set aside to cool slightly, at least 3 to 5 minutes. Using a spoon, scoop out the flesh from the cooked squash and transfer it to a blender or food processor. Add the cooked pears and purée until smooth. For younger babies, add enough water to reach the desired consistency. For

older children and adults, add salt, cinnamon, and orange zest, if using.

Roasted Squash with Maple Dressing

Special equipment: blender
Preparation: 5 minutes
Cooking: 40 minutes
Servings: 2 adults and 2 children

This is a great dish to make for babies who are transitioning to more solid foods, but who aren't really ready to chew hard foods or chunks. My younger daughter (who took a long, long time to start chewing solid foods) loved this dish, and we still make it on winter nights.

The taste-training element is in the dressing: the sweetness of the maple syrup and the acidity of the orange offsets the sage leaves, which pair wonderfully with the squash.

As with the recipe for Butternut Squash Purée on page 269, I've calculated adult servings, as I am assuming you'll want to enjoy this yummy dish along with your child!

1 large butternut squash
1 tablespoon salted butter or vegetable oil
1 teaspoon sea salt, optional

Maple Cinnamon Dressing:
60ml pure maple syrup
60ml orange juice
¼ teaspoon ground cinnamon
4 fresh sage leaves

1. Preheat the oven to 200°C/gas 6.
2. Halve the squash lengthwise and remove the seeds and strings. Rub the insides with butter. Place squash, cut-side down, in a baking dish with 60ml of water. Bake in the oven for 30 to 40 minutes, or until tender when pricked with a fork. Remove from the oven, sprinkle with salt, if using, and set aside to cool.
3. Meanwhile, make the Maple Cinnamon Sauce: In Dressing small saucepan over medium-low heat, combine the maple syrup, orange juice, and cinnamon and heat it gently for about 5 minutes. (Bonus: this will make your kitchen smell wonderful!) Set aside.
4. Make the crispy sage leaves: In a small pan over medium heat, melt the remaining butter. Add the whole sage leaves and sauté until they are browned and curl slightly at the edges, about 3 minutes. Transfer the leaves to a plate lined with a paper towel and set aside.
5. Using a spoon, scoop out the flesh from the cooked squash and transfer it to a blender. Add the maple syrup mixture and blend until smooth and creamy. Alternatively, for older kids and adults, you can serve the squash halves whole, with the maple cinnamon sauce served in a little bowl on the side so kids can drizzle it in the little "bowl" on top.
6. Serve warm, garnished with crispy sage leaves.

Squash Sage Soup

Special equipment: blender
Preparation: 10 minutes
Cooking: 50 minutes
Servings: 2 adults and 2 children

This is one of my all-time favorite soups. Depending on whether you like your soup sweet or savory, you can flavor it with either orange juice or *Brodo* (page 364) and orange juice. The baked garlic is so mellow that you barely notice it. The fried sage leaf garnish is a fun twist.

This soup freezes well, but make the crispy sage garnish right before serving.

2 small butternut squash, halved lengthwise and seeded
3 tablespoons olive oil
2 cloves garlic, halved (optional)
1 tablespoon salted butter
1 large onion, chopped
2 chopped fresh sage leaves plus 10 whole fresh sage leaves
720ml orange juice *or*
360ml *Brodo* (page 364) or ready-to-use low-sodium vegetable stock and 360ml orange juice, mixed
¼ teaspoon ground nutmeg
½ teaspoon dried thyme
1 teaspoon sea salt
½ teaspoon ground black pepper

1. Preheat the oven to 200°C/gas 6.
2. Brush the bottom of a baking dish and the cut surfaces of the squash with oil. Place half a clove of garlic inside each squash cavity and place the squash in the pan, cut-side down. Pour 120ml of water into the pan, cover with foil, and bake in the oven for 40 to 50 minutes, or until the squash is tender when pricked with a fork.
3. Meanwhile, in a small frying pan over medium heat, melt half of the butter. Add the onions and chopped sage, and cook until the onions turn golden brown, 4 to 5 minutes. Transfer the onion mixture to a plate and set aside.
4. Make the crispy sage leaves: In the same pan over

medium heat, melt the remaining butter. Add the whole sage leaves and sauté until they are browned and curl slightly at the edges, about 3 minutes. Transfer the crispy sage leaves to a plate lined with paper towel (to absorb excess butter) and set aside.

5. Using a spoon, scoop out the flesh from the cooked squash and transfer it to a blender. Add the cooked onions, garlic, if using, orange juice or *brodo* and orange juice, nutmeg, thyme, salt, and pepper and purée until smooth. Ladle into bowls and garnish with one or two crispy sage leaves. (I sometimes sprinkle salt on the crispy sage leaves right before using them as a garnish to make them extra tasty.)

Mild Thai Squash Curry

Special equipment: none
Preparation: 10 minutes
Cooking: 35 minutes
Servings: 4 adults or 6 children

Don't be alarmed by the word "curry"! I promise that this is a recipe even cautious children will love. The sweet coconut offsets the mild taste of the ginger. It's a wonderful introduction into the world of curries.

400g Thai rice (or 100g per adult or older child)
3 large carrots, peeled and cut into bite-size pieces
1 small acorn squash, peeled, halved, seeded, and cut into bite-size pieces
1 large sweet potato, peeled and cut into bite-size pieces
1 tablespoon vegetable oil
1 clove garlic, halved

4 small boneless, skinless chicken breasts, cut into bite-size pieces
400g can coconut milk
Juice of 1 lime (about 2 tablespoons)
½ teaspoon ground ginger
¼ teaspoon sea salt
1 teaspoon Thai curry paste
1 teaspoon liquid honey or packed dark brown sugar or pure maple syrup
15g finely chopped fresh coriander leaves

1. Set a medium saucepan over medium heat with 1 litre of water (for the rice) and a large saucepan over high heat with 2 litres of water (for the vegetables).
2. When the water in the medium saucepan is boiling, add the rice, reduce the heat to low, cover, and cook for 20 minutes, or as directed on the package. (The rice is cooked when fluffy and the water is fully absorbed.)
3. Meanwhile, in the other saucepan, add the carrots, squash, and sweet potato, reduce the heat to medium-high, and simmer until the vegetables are just tender, about 5 minutes. Drain the vegetables.
4. In a large frying pan over medium heat, heat the oil. Add the garlic and chicken and cook, stirring constantly, for 1 minute. Add the cooked carrots, squash, and sweet potato, the coconut milk, lime juice, ginger, salt, and Thai curry paste. Cover and simmer for 12 to 15 minutes, or until the vegetables are tender and the chicken is cooked through. Stir in the honey and coriander just before serving.

TOMATOES

A TOMATO PEACH
BASIL PUREE

B ROCK STAR RAGOUT

C PEEK-A-BOO
STUFFED TOMATOES

D TASTY TAGINE CASSEROLE

Tomato Peach Basil Purée
(a.k.a. Baby Gazpacho)

Special equipment: steamer insert (optional); food processor or blender
Preparation: 2 minutes
Cooking: 6 minutes
Servings: 6 to 8 baby jars or 1 adult

The flavors of tomato (which is, of course, a fruit) and peach are a wonderful blend. The slightly sweet taste of the peaches reduces the acidity of the tomatoes and lends a smooth creaminess to the purée. Bonus: this is the starting point for one of the world's best soups, Spanish gazpacho, a veggie-packed, super healthy, incredibly easy, no-cook cold summer soup. Think of it as the best veggie smoothie you ever tasted, and get ready to explore those tastes with your baby!

As with all of the other purée recipes, this makes a great adult soup, too. Double the recipe for each additional adult and garnish with a sprinkle of chopped basil.

This purée freezes well.

2 medium very ripe tomatoes, cored and chopped
1 or 2 fresh basil leaves, finely chopped
1 large or 2 small ripe peaches, pitted, peeled, and quartered

1. In a medium saucepan over medium-low heat, combine the tomatoes and basil with just enough water to cover the tomatoes. (The tomatoes will release more water while cooking.) Arrange the peaches on top of the tomatoes (so that they steam rather than boil—or they will get really mushy fast). Alternatively, steam the peaches in a separate saucepan using a steamer

insert. Cook until the peaches are soft, about 5 minutes. Strain the tomatoes and peaches, reserving the cooking liquid.

2. Using a food processor or blender, purée the tomatoes and peaches, adding enough cooking liquid to reach the desired consistency.

Taste-Training Tip: As your baby grows, you can gradually convert this soup into a gazpacho. Introducing one new ingredient at a time as you accustom your baby to the tastes, add these ingredients before blending: 240ml tomato juice, 75g chopped yellow or red pepper, 15g finely chopped fresh parsley leaves, 2 tablespoons olive oil plus 1 tablespoon lemon juice (or 30ml orange juice), ½ small chopped onion, 1 tablespoon chopped fresh basil leaves, ¼ teaspoon sea salt, and ¼ teaspoon ground black pepper. Experiment with the flavor combinations you like best!

Rockstar Ragout

Special equipment: food processor
Preparation: 5 minutes
Cooking: 15 minutes
Servings: 2 adults and 2 children (smallish servings)

Ragù is Italian comfort food. There's also a French version of this dish (a slow-cooked stew, often served with potatoes), but I prefer the Italian approach by far. There are many variations on this stew, but I like my version plain and simple. The French name (*ragoût*) comes from the (ancient) word *ragoûter,* which translates as "to revive the taste" or "to stimulate the appetite." This dish certainly does that!

If you have an older child who doesn't enjoy eating meat, try them on this melt-in-your-mouth dish. Serve it with pasta sprinkled with Parmesan. *Delicious!*

This dish freezes well.

1 tablespoon olive oil
1 clove garlic, halved
225g high-quality ground beef
2 carrots, peeled and sliced into 1.5-cm coins
2 x 400g cans chopped tomatoes
3 tablespoons tomato paste
½ teaspoon chopped fresh flat-leaf parsley leaves
¼ teaspoon dried thyme
¼ teaspoon dried oregano
Sea salt and ground black pepper, optional

1. In a medium saucepan over medium-low heat, heat the oil. Add the garlic and sauté for 1 minute, or until brown. Add the ground beef, increase the heat to medium-high, and cook, stirring continuously, for 1 minute. Add the carrots and cook, stirring occasionally, for 3 or 4 minutes, or until the beef is cooked through. Add the tomatoes, tomato paste, parsley, thyme, and oregano. Cover, reduce the heat to medium, and simmer for 10 minutes, stirring occasionally.

2. Transfer the beef mixture to a food processor and purée (see Note). For adults or older children, you might want to season with salt and pepper.

Taste-Training Note: For younger babies who aren't yet chewing, you can purée the mixture until smooth. You can progressively transition them to more solid textures by setting aside part of the beef mixture before puréeing, and then stirring it into the purée before serving. Make it progressively chunkier as your baby grows, and they'll be eating "grown-up" ragout in no time!

Peek-a-Boo Stuffed Tomatoes
(Tomates Farcies)

Special equipment: none
Preparation: 15 minutes
Cooking: 40 minutes
Servings: 4 adults or older children (as a side dish)

I couldn't resist including a readers' favorite recipe from *French Kids Eat Everything*. *Tomates farcies* are one of the most fun ways I know to serve tomatoes. They're stuffed with a savory ground beef mixture and then baked to perfection. The *farce* peeks out of the tomatoes in a coquettish sort of way; children love lifting up the tomato "hats" to see what lies underneath. Served with something that can absorb the delicious juices—rice and couscous are favorites—this is a nice, light, tasty meal.

2 tablespoons olive oil
1 small onion, minced
225g ground beef
4 large or 6 medium tomatoes
75g diced red or yellow pepper, optional
30g dried breadcrumbs
½ teaspoon dried parsley or oregano, optional
¼ teaspoon sea salt
¼ teaspoon ground black pepper
15g grated Parmesan cheese

1. Preheat the oven to 190°C/gas 5.
2. In a medium frying pan over low heat, heat the oil. Add the onion and sauté until golden brown, about 5 minutes. Increase the heat to medium-high, add the

ground beef, and cook, stirring continuously, for 2 minutes or until lightly browned. Reduce the heat to medium-low and sauté until the beef is cooked through, 6 to 8 minutes.

3. Meanwhile, prepare the tomatoes: Slice off the tops and set them aside, then, using a small spoon or melon baller, hollow out the insides of the tomatoes, transferring the pulp to a bowl. (The result will look like little bowls.) Arrange the tomatoes upside down on a plate and set aside to allow the juice to drain. Chop the reserved tomato pulp and add it to the simmering beef mixture along with the red pepper, if using.

4. In a small bowl, combine the breadcrumbs, herbs, and salt and pepper. (You can try out any herbs and spices you like—my sister-in-law uses paprika. Get creative!) Add the breadcrumb mixture to the beef mixture and stir well to combine.

5. Spoon the meat mixture (the "*farce*") into the tomato "bowls" and sprinkle with Parmesan. Put the tops back on the tomatoes. Transfer the stuffed tomatoes to a baking dish and bake in the oven for 20 to 25 minutes, or until they are deliciously melt-in-your-mouth. Remove from the oven and cool for 5 minutes before serving.

Note: This dish can easily be prepared the night before and refrigerated until ready to bake. If you put the tomatoes straight into the oven from the fridge, you'll need to increase the baking time to 25 or 30 minutes.

Taste-Testing Tip: For younger babies still getting used to solid foods, you can combine about ⅓ of a cooked tomato with some meat mixture, tomato paste, and a little water, and purée for a ready-to-eat ragout.

Tasty Tagine Casserole

Special equipment: none
Preparation: 5 minutes
Cooking: 20 minutes
Servings: 2 adults and 2 children

A tagine is a North African vegetable stew—eaten everywhere, in endlessly delicious variations (sort of like Asian stir-fries). This simple dish combines the savory flavor of meat (chicken) with sweet raisins and spices. It's another great dish to encourage reluctant meat-eaters, as the chicken is melt-in-your-mouth tender. *Yum!*

2 tablespoons olive oil
4 skinless boneless chicken breasts, cut into bite-size pieces
1 small onion, diced
1 clove garlic, halved
¼ teaspoon ground ginger
¼ teaspoon ground allspice
½ teaspoon ground cinnamon
¼ teaspoon ground turmeric, optional
¼ teaspoon ground cumin, optional
4 carrots, peeled and cut into bite-size pieces
1 large zucchini, peeled and cut into bite-size pieces
2 large tomatoes, chopped
1 tablespoon tomato paste
120ml orange juice
70g sultanas
Sea salt and ground black pepper, optional
Cooked rice, polenta, couscous, or quinoa, for serving
Chopped fresh flat-leaf parsley leaves, optional

1. In a large saucepan over medium heat, heat the oil. Increase the heat to high, add the chicken, and cook, stirring often, until lightly seared, 3 to 4 minutes each side. Reduce the heat to medium, add the onion, garlic, ginger, allspice, cinnamon, and turmeric and cumin, if using, and cook for 3 minutes, until the onion is just starting to turn golden brown. Add the carrots, zucchini, tomatoes, tomato paste, orange juice, and 120ml of water. Increase the heat to high and bring the stew to a boil. Once boiling, cover, reduce the heat to low, and simmer for 10 minutes, stirring occasionally.

2. Add the sultanas and salt and pepper, if using, and cook for 2 to 3 minutes, uncovered, until the sauce reduces slightly (it will still be quite watery). Serve with your desired grain or starch, sprinkled with parsley for a bit of color.

Taste-Training Tip: For smaller babies, purée a morsel or two of chicken with some carrots and a little of the sauce from the finished dish.

ZUCCHINI

(A) SOFT-AS-A-CLOUD
PUREE

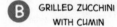

(B) GRILLED ZUCCHINI
WITH CUMIN

(C) ZUCCHINI FLAN

(D) ZUCCHINI QUICHE

Melt-in-your-mouth Zucchini Purée

This soft-as-a-cloud purée is one of the simplest purées of all to make for your baby (and is often used as a starter purée in France). The texture is indescribably light and airy. For younger babies, you can serve this plain. For older babies (9 months and up), start experimenting by adding a little bit of cumin or allspice—just a pinch at first!

Special equipment: food processor or blender
Preparation: 2 minutes
Cooking: 5 minutes
Servings: 4 to 6 baby jars (depending on the size of your zucchini)

2 medium zucchini, peeled and cut into 5-cm chunks
1 teaspoon salted butter
Pinch ground allspice or ground cumin, optional

1. Bring a medium saucepan half-filled with water to a boil over high heat. Add the zucchini, reduce the heat to medium-low, and simmer for 5 minutes, or until the zucchini is tender. Strain the zucchini, reserving the cooking liquid.
2. Using a food processor or blender, purée the zucchini until smooth, adding enough cooking liquid to reach the desired consistency. Serve dabbed with butter.

I made the zucchini purée today and my 8-month-old devoured it! Her first taste of the big Z!
—Brandy

Roasted Zucchini with Cumin

Special equipment: none
Preparation: 5 minutes
Cooking: 10 minutes
Servings: 2 adults and 2 kids (as side dish)

When your child is ready to chew solid foods, this is a fun way to introduce them to roasted vegetables. The zucchini will become soft and tender in the oven, and the flavors of cumin and olive oil marry beautifully. (You can also cook these on the grill, but the oven version is tender and easier for children to chew.)

This also makes a nice adult side dish; just pop a few extra zucchini in the oven!

1 large zucchini
1 clove garlic, halved, optional
1 teaspoon ground cumin
1 teaspoon sea salt, optional
2 tablespoons olive oil

1. Preheat the oven to 200°C/gas 6.
2. Using a paring knife, peel the zucchini and remove the ends (no need to peel for adults), then cut them in half lengthwise. Make shallow criss-cross incisions across the cut sides of the zucchini and lay them, cut-side up, in a baking dish.
3. If using garlic, rub the halved clove over the cut side of the zucchini. Sprinkle with cumin and salt, if using (careful, you will need very little salt in this dish). Drizzle with oil. Add 120ml of water to the baking dish. Bake in the oven for 5 minutes, flip zucchini

over, and bake 5 minutes more, or until desired tenderness.

I made the roasted zucchini tonight. I could not believe how tasty it was. So simple and so good! My 2½-year-old ate it without much encouragement. I will definitely make it again. It was great. I may even try it with the skin on next time!

—Babette

Zucchini Flan

Special equipment: box grater; 20-cm round baking dish
Preparation: 15 minutes plus 10 minutes for cooling
Cooking: 45 minutes
Servings: 6 adults (as a side dish)

Flans are a great way to introduce children to the taste of baked eggs so they can move on to enjoying quiche with the whole family.

This simple recipe highlights the mild taste of the zucchini and combines it with onions that have been cooked until mild, rich, and melt-in-your-mouth. The added touch of cumin prepares your child for the more complex taste of curries in other dishes.

2 tablespoons salted butter
2 tablespoons olive oil
1 medium onion, very finely sliced
½ teaspoon ground nutmeg
5 or 6 fresh basil leaves, very finely chopped
Sea salt and ground black pepper, optional

4 medium zucchini, peeled and cut into 3mm coins
1 teaspoon ground cumin
3 large eggs
160ml whipping cream or ricotta cheese
60g grated Cheddar cheese
30g grated Parmesan cheese

1. Preheat the oven to 200°C/gas 6. Grease a baking dish with 1 tablespoon butter.
2. In a medium saucepan over medium heat, heat 1 tablespoon oil. Add 1 tablespoon butter, the onion, nutmeg, basil, and a pinch of salt, if using, and stir to combine. Cover and cook for 6 to 7 minutes, stirring occasionally, until the onions are tender.
3. Meanwhile, in a large frying pan over medium-high heat, heat the remaining 1 tablespoon oil. Add the zucchini, sprinkle it with cumin, and cook for 5 minutes, stirring often, until just tender (do not overcook!). Remove from the heat, drain any excess water, and sprinkle with salt and pepper, if using.
4. In a medium bowl, whisk together the eggs and cream. Set aside.
5. In the prepared baking dish, spread half the cooked onions in an even layer. Top with half the cooked zucchini, then half the cheese. Repeat the three layers with the remaining ingredients. Pour the egg mixture over the top, ensuring everything is evenly covered. (Cheese lovers might want to sprinkle a little extra Parmesan on top.) Bake in the oven for 30 minutes, or until the vegetables are cooked through and the cheese is melted and browned. Remove from the oven and set aside to cool for 5 to 10 minutes. (This dish stays very hot in the center, and resting the flan will help the pieces slide out more easily.) To serve, cut the flan into slices.

Quick Zucchini-Ham Quiche

Special equipment: box grater; 25-cm pie dish
Preparation: 7 minutes
Cooking: 40 minutes
Serving: 2 adults and 2 children (with two second helpings!)

Easy and quick to make, this no-crust version of classic French quiche will please adults and children alike. Quiche is also versatile, as it can be eaten hot or cold, for lunch or for dinner, and with any combination of vegetables that you can think of.

This is a children's version of the recipe—it uses more milk and fewer eggs than a quiche intended for adults. The resulting dish is fluffier, less dense, and less eggy, and so more likely to please young palates. For older children and adults, reduce the milk by 120ml and add 1 more egg (or play with the ratio of eggs and milk until you find the texture your family prefers).

10 large eggs
120ml milk
½ teaspoon ground nutmeg
1 teaspoon ground cumin
Sea salt and ground black pepper, optional
115g grated Gruyére (preferred) or Cheddar cheese
225g cubed cooked ham or 115g crumbled cooked bacon
1 medium zucchini, peeled and grated

1. Preheat the oven to 190°C/gas 5. Grease a pie dish.
2. In a large bowl, beat the eggs lightly, then add the milk, nutmeg, and cumin and mix well. Add a pinch of salt and pepper, if using. Stir in the cheese, then the ham and zucchini.
3. Pour the mixture into the prepared pie plate and bake

in the oven for 30 to 40 minutes, or until a knife slid into the center comes out clean. Remove from the oven and set aside for 5 minutes to cool before serving (the quiche will settle, and you'll be able to cut it more neatly).

Taste-Training Tip: Changing your quiche ingredients is a great way to introduce new vegetables. The reassuringly familiar look of the dish will likely entice even the wariest of eaters to try a new, yummy vegetable. Once your child likes this version, try quiche with red peppers or even broccoli!

The flavor is quite subtle, but for a quick weeknight meal you can't go wrong with that. I served it to my husband and 2-year-old, and then proceeded to have a 15-minute uninterrupted conversation with my husband while my daughter quietly ate hers. She was hungry and it hit the spot! Love that! All in all, a hit.

—Teresa

Fun with Flavors! Fruit Recipes

APPLES

A SPICE IS NICE PURÉE

B BABIES' BAKED APPLES

C SARAH'S SLAW SALAD

D CURRIED APPLE SOUP

Spice Is Nice Purée

Special equipment: blender or food processor
Preparation: 5 minutes
Cooking: 5 minutes
Servings: 6 to 8 baby jars

Most babies love apples in any form, so they're a great medium for introducing other flavors. In this purée, a little hint of ginger is combined with the teensiest bit of cinnamon. If desired, you can start with just cinnamon, or just ginger, instead of using both spices as called for in the recipe. Baby will get used to more variety and hopefully be more interested in the curry dishes you'll serve when they're older!

This recipe freezes well.

4 apples, peeled, cored, and quartered (see Note)
¼ teaspoon ground cinnamon
Tiny pinch dried ginger
½ teaspoon fresh lemon juice, optional
Plain yogurt, for serving, optional

1. In a medium saucepan over medium-low heat, bring 240ml of water to a boil. Add the apples, cover, and simmer until soft, 4 to 5 minutes. Strain the apples, reserving the cooking liquid. Transfer the cooked apples to a blender or food processor, add the cinnamon and ginger, and purée. If you prefer a thinner purée, slowly add enough cooking liquid to reach the desired consistency. If you prefer a tangier taste, add the lemon juice. Be sure to let the purée cool before serving—it will be hot! The purée is lovely with a little dollop of yogurt for a nice texture contrast.

Note: In this recipe, I prefer using sweeter apples such as Gala or Pink Lady. Granny Smith or other sour apples don't work as well.

Babies' Baked Apples

Special equipment: none
Preparation: 10 minutes
Cooking: 30 minutes
Servings: 1 apple per person

This dish is a reader favorite from *French Kids Eat Everything*. It's one of our favorite wintertime desserts and a real time-saver. I pop the apples in the oven before I start making dinner, and by the time the meal is ready to serve, the smell of the apples fills the house, beckoning the children to the table (at least, that's the theory!).

This recipe can be used to help transition babies to more solid foods. Baked long enough, the texture of the apple is as creamy as applesauce. Reduce the baking time, and the consistency gets progressively more solid.

1 apple per person, washed, stemmed, and cored, skin pricked with a fork
1 teaspoon pure maple syrup per apple, plus more for drizzling (see Note)
Ground cinnamon, optional

1. Preheat the oven to 190°C/gas 5.
2. Arrange the apples upright in a baking dish and add 120ml of water to the dish. Drizzle maple syrup into the hole in each apple (a little may seep out of the bottom). Dust with cinnamon, if using.
3. Bake the apples in the oven for about 25 to 30

minutes, or until they reach a desired consistency. Just before serving, baste the apples with the sauce in the bottom of the dish. Serve the apples on individual plates, with maple syrup drizzled around the top of the apples or sprinkled with a bit of sugar and cinnamon.

Safety Tip: Be sure to remove the apples from the oven at least 5 minutes before you plan to eat them. They stay piping hot inside and can burn little tongues. Don't rely on the heat of the outside of the apple to judge whether it's safe to serve; the flesh inside will remain much hotter than the outside surface, which will cool down quite quickly. We cut the apples for our children and let the pieces cool on plates on the counter before bringing them to the table.

Note: To make this as the French do, substitute 1 tablespoon sugar and 1 tablespoon melted butter for the maple syrup. If using the butter/sugar combination, spoon it into the apple cores after they've been baking for about 15 minutes.

I made the baked apples last night for the toddlers and the rest of my family, and they were a huge hit with everyone! The apples were delicious on their own, but we made it a party and added a scoop of vanilla ice cream! I have a feeling I'll be making this all winter long.

—Meg

Sarah's Slaw Salad

Special equipment: food processor
Preparation: 15 minutes
Cooking: none
Servings: 2 adults and 2 to 4 children (as a side salad)

I created this recipe for Sarah, one of the more reluctant kids who taste tested the recipes in this book with me. It's a great way to introduce children to coleslaw: it uses apples, carrots, and only a small amount of cabbage (at first). The oil and vinegar dressing is a lighter alternative to the rich, creamy dressings often used in coleslaws. This salad also subtly introduces a new spice (cumin) that's one of the key ingredients in curry—preparing kids' taste buds for the curried soup that follows in this series.

2 apples, peeled, cored, and cut into bite-size pieces (I prefer Granny Smith)
1 tablespoon fresh lemon juice
75g raisins or currants, soaked in 240ml warm water, optional
¼ purple (red) cabbage, finely sliced
2 large carrots, peeled and finely grated

Dressing:
3 tablespoons extra virgin olive oil
1 tablespoon balsamic vinegar or apple cider vinegar
½ teaspoon sea salt
¼ teaspoon ground cumin, optional
⅛ teaspoon ground cinnamon, optional

Toppings:
1 shallot, minced
1 tablespoon roasted sunflower seeds, optional
1 tablespoon minced fresh mint or parsley leaves or 1 teaspoon dried mint or parsley

1. In a bowl, combine the apples with the lemon juice to prevent browning.
2. If using the raisins, drain using a fine-mesh sieve, discarding the soaking water, and transfer to a large bowl. Add the cabbage, carrots, and prepared apples and mix to combine.

3. Make the dressing: In a small bowl, whisk together the oil, vinegar, salt, and cumin and cinnamon, if using. (Note: the quantity of dressing is deliberately small, so that the salad is not overdressed. If you know you like this dressing, you can double the quantities.)

4. Add the dressing to the salad and toss to coat well. Sprinkle with your toppings of choice. Serve at room temperature or slightly chilled.

Taste-Training Tips: For kids who are still learning to like some of these foods, try this: announce a "buffet salad" starter for your meal and place small bowls of each sliced ingredient on the counter or table. Kids can serve themselves from each bowl and "mix" their own salad. The only rules are that a) they have to take something from each bowl, and b) they have to taste everything they've taken. This will give kids who balk at certain fruits or vegetables the sense of control they might be seeking, while still encouraging them to taste new things.

Start with the small amount of cabbage as per the recipe, but as the kids begin (hopefully) to like it, increase the amount of red cabbage gradually, until it is equal to the carrot.

My very picky 3-year-old son ate his entire portion and did not complain one bit! He didn't seem to mind the new taste of the cabbage. The entire thing was so easy and quick to put together—it took 10 minutes from start to finish. Will be going in our repertoire!

—Jessica

Curried Apple Soup

Special equipment: food processor or blender
Preparation: 10 minutes
Cooking: 20 minutes
Servings: 2 adults and 2 children

Before I had children, curried apple-squash soup was one of my favorites. So when I started introducing curry spices to my children, this seemed like the natural go-to dish. I've simplified it for busy parents but preserved the essence: sweet apples offset the savory soup with a hint of mild curry. After trial and error, I found that this works best with juicy, tart apples (such as Spartan or Granny Smith). The flavors in this soup will intensify if made a few hours prior to the meal (or even the night before).

This is a great lunch soup; just pack it in thermoses and go! I also make large batches and freeze them in quantities appropriate for one family meal. Then I simply remove what I need from the freezer in the morning; by dinnertime, the soup is thawed and ready to be gently heated and enjoyed!

1 tablespoon butter
1 tablespoon olive oil
3 tablespoons chopped onion or leek, white part only
1 large sweet potato, peeled and chopped
100g chopped celery or celeriac
200g peeled, cored, chopped apples
1 to 2 teaspoons curry powder, to taste
½ teaspoon ground ginger or 1 teaspoon freshly grated ginger-root
1 litre *Brodo* (page 364) or ready-to-use low-sodium vegetable or chicken stock
2 bay leaves

1 teaspoon sea salt, optional
240ml reduced-fat cream (for a rich soup) or whole milk (for a lighter soup)

1. In a large saucepan over medium-low heat, melt the butter in the olive oil. Add the onion and celery and sauté for 5 minutes. Add the apples, sweet potato, curry powder, and ginger, reduce the heat to medium, and sauté for 3 minutes, until the apples are just tender. Add the *brodo,* bay leaves, and salt, if using. Increase heat to high and bring to a boil. Once boiling, reduce the heat to medium and simmer until the celery is tender, 6 to 8 minutes. Remove from heat. Discard the bay leaves.
2. Using a food processor or blender, purée the soup. Return the soup to the pot, if necessary, then stir in the cream. Taste and add more salt, if desired. Reheat the soup if necessary—but *gently* (don't let it boil).

Serving Tip: After pouring the soup into bowls, swirl in a small spoonful of cream, sour cream, or plain yogurt, or sprinkle with a small pinch of dried thyme or mint for a decorative effect.

The flavor of this soup is out of this world—it could be served in a five-star restaurant. I was worried that my husband would freak out about this recipe, as he never likes fruit in his savory food. Well . . . he loved *it.*
                                                          —*Babette*

AVOCADO

Amazing Avocado Smoothie

Special equipment: blender or food processor
Preparation: 5 minutes
Cooking: none
Servings: 2 adults and 2 children

Rich, satisfying, and super-nutritious, avocados are a quick and easy go-to option for parents. Although we tend to think of avocados as ingredients in savory dishes (such as guacamole), they're often served sweetened in other parts of the world (avocado ice cream!). Avocado's versatility makes it a great base from which to introduce your child to lots of different flavors and textures.

This smoothie is easy to make in the mornings and has now become a family breakfast favorite on schooldays. My kids love peeling the bananas and taking turns deciding what fruit to add. For cautious or reactive eaters, this can actually be a useful strategy: they'll be more willing to try "their" creation. You can enjoy this thick (eat it with a spoon!) or thin (sip it through a straw), as desired, by varying the amounts of liquids you add.

240ml fruit juice
120ml water
1 avocado, peeled and pitted (see Note)
1 ripe banana
Juice of ½ lemon (about 1 tablespoon)
1 fresh peach, cubed, optional

1. In a blender or food processor, combine the juice, water, avocado, banana, lemon juice, and peach, if using, and purée until smooth.

Note: Avocado can sometimes have a slightly bitter aftertaste if really ripe, so I don't use overly ripe avocados. If you do, you might want to add a teaspoon of maple syrup or another ½ banana. Don't skip the lemon juice: avocado needs something acidic for balance.

Taste-Training Tip: Be inventive with this recipe. Try 360ml of orange juice (skip the lemon juice) plus 120ml plain yogurt. Part of the fun for kids is seeing how different ingredients result in different textures and tastes, so let them experiment, too! My kids have managed to make only one or two undrinkable smoothies, and their experiments were always interesting. Note, though, that berries don't work very well in this recipe—at least not according to our daughters and the test families!

Peeling avocados is easy. Using a sharp knife, cut the avocado lengthwise through the skin, all the way to the pit, all the way around. You now have two halves, still stuck together. Hold each half and twist in opposite directions. It should separate easily, and you will be able to lift one half off. The pit will remain in the other half. Whack the pit carefully with the sharp edge of the knife (so that it "bites" into the pit) and then lift the pit out. While the skin is still on, slice (or dice) the avocado flesh, then scoop it out with a spoon. (You can also find some good videos online that explain this technique.)

Beginner's Guacamole

Special equipment: food processor (optional)
Preparation: 5 minutes
Cooking: none
Servings: 2 baby jars

Guacamole is a great dish for kids—packed full of healthy veggies—and it's probably one of the easiest recipes in this book. Start off by serving plain avocado to your baby (directly out of the avocado using a spoon is the easiest way). You can then start adding the ingredients below, one by one, until baby is eating something that fairly closely resembles adult guacamole. See the stages listed below for three versions for children of increasing ages.

We usually double this recipe to make a small side dish for our family.

1 ripe avocado
1 tablespoon sour cream or yogurt
¼ teaspoon orange or lime juice
50g finely diced tomato
1 tablespoon finely diced fresh coriander leaves
¼ teaspoon ground cumin
1 tablespoon finely minced red or yellow onion

Stage 1: Serve the avocado plain or, for older babies (1 year or older), serve half an avocado on a plate, with the little "bowl" (made by removing the pit) filled with a dip or dressing that they like. I use the Classic Vinaigrette (page 365); the mild acidity perfectly offsets the rich, creamy avocado taste.

Stage 2: Peel and pit the avocado (see previous page). In a food processor, combine the avocado with the sour cream and orange juice and purée.

Stage 3: Follow Stage 2 above, then add the tomato. Once your child likes this version, add the coriander. Once that has been accepted, add the cumin. Finish with the minced onion. *Voilà:* guacamole!

Taste-Training Tip: If you have children at different stages, you can also place these ingredients in separate bowls on the table and invite the kids to mix their own guacamole. Adventurous eaters will use more ingredients, and kids who are still learning to like this dish will experience some low-pressure positive peer encouragement as they see the others trying and enjoying the various ingredients.

I really loved the idea of using the avocado as a bowl, so I just chopped up tomatoes and coriander and served it with a vinaigrette. At first my 3-year-old said it was "yucky," but then he tried it—the big hurdle being getting him to put the salsa and avocado on the spoon and eat it all at the same time. It got a "yummy"!

—Martha

Awesome Avocado Ice Pops

Special equipment: food processor; ice-pop trays
Preparation: 5 minutes plus at least 2 hours for freezing
Cooking: none
Servings: at least 6 big (double) ice pops

Ice pops are an amazing way to introduce new flavors to your kids. We enjoy them throughout the summer (and homemade ones are so much cheaper than store-bought!). This recipe is adapted from Fany Gerson's *Paletas* cookbook, which features tropical ice pops and shaved ice inspired by the flavors of Mexico and includes everything from tamarind and hibiscus flower to strawberry. If this recipe inspires you, her cookbook is a great next step.

1 large ripe avocado, halved, pitted, and peeled
80ml grape or apple juice
80ml coconut milk

2 tablespoons fresh lime juice
Pinch sea salt
40g berries, optional

1. In a food processor, combine the avocado, fruit juice, coconut milk (do not use coconut cream!), lime juice, salt, berries, if using, and 80ml of water and purée. Pour into an ice-pop mold and freeze.

Avocado Salsa Salad

Special equipment: none
Preparation: 10 minutes
Cooking: none
Servings: 2 adults and 2 children (with lots of leftovers)

This is a tasty and slightly unusual texture combination that is also super-good for you: research has shown that adding avocado to salads and/or salsa can increase your intake of nutrients. This is because some nutrients are fat-soluble, and avocados have a relatively high proportion of (healthy) fats (in fact, they're one of the only fruits that do).

This is a great summer salad recipe, with contrasting colors and textures. On hot days, we sometimes eat this with bread as our main meal at lunchtime.

2 ripe but still firm avocados, halved, pitted, peeled, and cut into 2.5-cm cubes
2 tablespoons fresh lime juice
1 tablespoon minced fresh coriander leaves, optional
¼ teaspoon sea salt
1 small head romaine or green leaf lettuce, torn into bite-size pieces

½ red or green pepper, cored, seeded, and diced
½ small red onion, finely diced
4 ripe plum tomatoes, chopped, or 12 cherry tomatoes, halved
30g sunflower seeds, optional
1 tablespoon extra virgin olive oil

1. In a small bowl, combine the avocados with 1 tablespoon of the lime juice and the coriander, if using. Season with salt and set aside.
2. In a large bowl, combine the lettuce, red pepper, onion, tomatoes, and sunflower seeds, if using. Add the remaining 1 tablespoon of lime juice and the olive oil and toss to combine. Just before serving, spoon the avocado mixture on top of the salad and *lightly* toss to combine (this will keep the avocado from getting mushy).

Taste-Training Tip: For toddlers or older kids reluctant to eat salad, try making sure they get smaller pieces of lettuce on their plate. Some kids start with the "crunchy" parts of lettuce leaves (the central spine of the leaf), which seem to be easier to chew than the more floppy, textured ends of the leaves.

BERRIES

A ROCKIN' RED GRANITA

B BLACKBERRY SUPER SALAD

C PERFECT BLUEBERRY PARFAIT

D SWEET & SOUR BLUEBERRY
GLAZED CHICKEN

Rockin' Red Granita

Special equipment: food processor
Preparation: 10 minutes plus 1 hour for freezing
Cooking: 5 minutes
Servings: 6 adults or children

Raspberries are a wonderful fruit for introducing tangy flavors to children. Their sweetness is naturally offset by just a hint of acidity—a little "zing" that adds a nice touch to this dish. The recipe also uses tomatoes, which are technically a fruit. The tomatoes balance out the sweetness of the raspberries (and they're much cheaper, making this a reasonably priced berry dish; just make sure the tomatoes are ripe).

This recipe is served cold, which will be a new experience for many babies. It's perfect for a hot summer day. Think of this as a healthy equivalent to sorbet for little ones!

115g raspberries
225g ripe tomatoes, chopped
60ml peach or apple fruit juice
2 teaspoons finely chopped fresh mint leaves
6 to 8 whole fresh mint leaves, for garnish

1. In a food processor, lightly process the raspberries, tomatoes, fruit juice, and chopped mint (see Note).
2. Transfer the berry mixture to a small saucepan over medium heat and simmer for 5 minutes, stirring constantly. Divide the mixture evenly among 6 small bowls and set aside to cool (you can also freeze it in one large container, but it may take longer). Once cooled, freeze for about 45 minutes to 1 hour, stirring

a few times, until just frozen. Using a fork or spoon, break up the granita. Garnish with mint leaves and serve. If you have extra raspberries, use them as a garnish.

Note: Smaller babies will need the granita to be very smooth; older babies may prefer it slightly chunky. For younger babies, you may want to strain the mixture through a fine-mesh sieve to remove the tomato seeds (I don't bother doing this).

I took a bite and thought, This is different. Maybe I don't like this. *But then I took a second bite, and I couldn't stop eating it. I finished my serving!*
—Sarah, age 8

Blackberry Super Salad

Special equipment: none
Preparation: 10 minutes plus 1 hour for chilling
Cooking: none
Servings: 2 adults and 2 children

This is a fun take on a fruit salad that can be served as a starter or dessert. The ginger gives it a little bit of bite that is offset by the fruit. It's a fun way to introduce your kids to "sharp" tastes. The thyme is an interesting contrast with the sweetness of the fruit and the spiciness of the ginger. This will be an unusual set of flavors for most children, so don't be surprised if they say "I don't like it" at first. It usually means "I don't know it yet." For more reluctant eaters, the honey syrup will help make things go a little more smoothly. Don't give up on the first try!

Honey Syrup:
1 tablespoon liquid honey or pure maple syrup or granulated sugar
120ml water

Salad:
4 fresh, ripe peaches and/or nectarines, pitted, peeled, and chopped
70g blackberries or blueberries
1 teaspoon minced fresh thyme leaves
1 teaspoon grated lemon zest
2 tablespoons fresh lemon juice
½ teaspoon grated fresh gingerroot, optional

1. To make the Honey Syrup (optional): In a small saucepan over medium-high heat, combine the honey and water and bring it to a boil. Reduce the heat to medium-low and simmer until the liquid is reduced by half, about 10 minutes. Remove from the heat and set aside to cool.
2. In a large bowl, combine the peaches and blackberries. Add the honey syrup, if using, then add the thyme, lemon zest and juice, and ginger, if using. Stir gently to combine (don't overmix!). Refrigerate for 1 hour before serving.

Taste-Training Tip: If you're introducing ginger to your child for the first time, set aside a portion of this salad without the ginger and serve that first. If your child likes it, then offer them the ginger option. Ask your child about the taste of ginger: is it spicy but sweet? How does it feel on their tongue?

Fun with Ginger

This is a great activity to do with your child! Investigate the smell and taste of fresh gingerroot. Your child will be intrigued by how mild it smells from the outside, but how spicy it tastes when it's peeled and sliced. For more reluctant kids, try first giving them something else with ginger (ginger cookies, gingerbread, candied ginger), and then ask them to taste the fresh ginger to see if they can detect a similar flavor. Research shows that children are more likely to accept new flavors if they're introduced to the sources first. This is about taste familiarization, not actually eating the ginger, so please do this activity at a time and place not associated with a meal.

Perfect Blueberry Parfait

Special equipment: 4 to 6 small, thin juice glasses
Preparation: 5 minutes
Cooking: none
Servings: 2 adults and 2 children

This layered dessert recipe is an adaptation of a popular French tactic for quick, easy, yet visually enticing aperitifs or desserts: *verrines*. *Verre* means "glass" in French, and a *verrine* means "little glass"—usually a thin glass that shows off the layers nicely. The French get really creative: for example, avocado might be layered with shrimp or crab mousse and topped with bits of candied citrus. The layers are much thinner than in the classic North American parfait and look more elegant (in my opinion!).

In this easy *verrine* recipe, the combination of blueberries and walnuts may seem a little odd, but that's the point: the moist, sweet blueberries are a nice complement to the dry, earthy flavor of the nuts. Note that a full-fat yogurt, such as Greek yogurt, works best to hold the layers.

Kids love helping to put this dessert together. It's quick and easy to prepare, and looks festive and fun. Perfect!

280g fresh or frozen blueberries
480ml plain, vanilla, or raspberry Greek yogurt
90g walnuts, chopped
4 teaspoons granola, optional

1. If using frozen blueberries, microwave them on high in a microwave-safe bowl for about 60 seconds, or until the juices just start flowing. If using fresh blueberries, place them in a small saucepan with a tiny bit of water and simmer over medium-high heat for 2 to 3 minutes until just tender; cool before using.
2. Spoon a thin layer (about 2 tablespoons) of yogurt into each small glass. Top with a thin layer of blueberries. Add alternating layers of yogurt and blueberries until you're near the top. Finish with a layer of walnuts and granola, if using (great for breakfast!), and garnish with a few blueberries.

We ate this for breakfast! Our usual school morning breakfast is either a fried or hard-boiled egg, a piece of toast with either honey or apple butter, and a yogurt parfait. It's actually very fast! The girls never tire of the presentation.

—Lori

Sweet and Sour Blueberry-Glazed Chicken

Special equipment: none
Preparation: 10 minutes
Cooking: 30 minutes
Servings: 2 adults and 2 children

Chicken is often a family favorite, but it's easy to fall into a bit of a routine (nuggets, anyone?). This is a fun way to expand your children's repertoire: the sauce is just sweet enough to please most palates and contrasts nicely with the chicken. Bonus: the cooked chicken is moist, which will enable some kids who are resistant to chicken to really enjoy this dish.

2 tablespoons butter
2 tablespoons olive oil
4 boneless skinless chicken breasts or 675g skinless chicken legs
Sea salt and ground black pepper, to taste

Sweet and Sour Blueberry Glaze:
30g sliced onion or shallots
140g fresh or frozen blueberries, plus extra for garnish
80ml balsamic vinegar
60ml pure maple syrup or Honey Syrup (page 309)
1 tablespoon chopped fresh rosemary or 1½ teaspoons dried rosemary
1 sprig fresh rosemary, for garnish
1 teaspoon fresh lemon juice, optional
½ teaspoon sea salt
¼ teaspoon ground black pepper

1. Preheat the oven to 190°C/gas 5.
2. In a large frying pan over medium-high heat, melt 1

tablespoon butter in 1 tablespoon oil. Season the chicken with salt and pepper, to taste. When the butter mixture is hot (sputtering!), add the chicken and sear for 1 minute or until light golden brown, then flip and sear the other side. Transfer the chicken to a baking dish and set aside.

3. To the same frying pan over medium-high heat, melt the remaining 1 tablespoon butter in the remaining 1 tablespoon oil. Stir in the onions and cook until softened and translucent, 4 to 5 minutes. Add the blueberries, increase the heat to high, and cook for 2 minutes. Reduce the heat to medium and stir in the vinegar, maple syrup, and rosemary and season with ½ teaspoon salt and ¼ teaspoon pepper. Simmer for 10 minutes, or until the blueberries start to dissolve. (For a more tart sauce with a real "zing," add the lemon juice.)

4. Pour the blueberry mixture over the prepared chicken and bake in the oven for 15 to 20 minutes, or until the chicken is cooked through. Serve garnished with a sprig of fresh rosemary and dotted with blueberries, if desired.

This was a breakthrough: the first time our 8-year-old girl ate non-nugget, unbreaded chicken. As always, she liked the sweetness. My wife and I also really liked the flavor mix of the maple syrup, blueberries, and balsamic.

—Jon

CANTALOUPE

B CANTALOUPE COMPOTE

C CHILLED CANTALOUPE GINGER SOUP

D SUMMER CANTALOUPE SALAD

Cantaloupe Compote

Special equipment: blender
Preparation: 5 minutes
Cooking: none
Servings: 6 to 8 baby jars

Melon is often a kids' favourite, and makes for a wonderful dessert. This compote is deliciously simple. When you serve cantaloupe to adults and older children (perhaps for a summer dessert), you can whip this up for baby.

This compote freezes well.

1 small ripe cantaloupe (see Note)

1. Using a sharp knife, cut the melon in half and, using a spoon, scoop out the seeds (discard seeds). Slice each half lengthwise to make "smile" (crescent) shapes. Cut the rind from each slice, then cut the slices into smaller chunks.
2. Transfer the cantaloupe to a blender and blend until smooth (it'll blend into a nice compote without the need for added liquid).

Note: A cantaloupe is ripe when it's pinkish-yellow rather than green and you can smell a fruity odor at the stem end.

Taste-Training Tip: Cantaloupe pairs wonderfully with raspberries and lemon or lime juice. As baby grows older, try experimenting with these flavor combinations!

Chilled Cantaloupe Ginger Soup

On those summer days when it's too hot to cook, chilled soups are a great choice: quick to make, hydrating, refreshing. In fact, they're just a thin version of fruit smoothies, so you could always call this a smoothie. But the addition of basil and yogurt makes this creamy enough that I consider it a soup. You say *potayto*, I say *potahto*!

Special equipment: blender
Preparation: 5 minutes
Cooking: none
Servings: 6 adults/older children

1 small ripe cantaloupe (see Note)
120ml plain Greek yogurt
⅛ teaspoon ground ginger
Juice of 1 lime (about 2 tablespoons)
1 teaspoon liquid honey
2 or 3 fresh mint leaves or 1 tablespoon dried mint
2 or 3 fresh basil leaves or 1 tablespoon dried basil
Pinch sea salt

1. Using a sharp knife, cut the melon in half and, using a spoon, scoop out the seeds (discard seeds). Slice each half lengthwise to make "smile" (crescent) shapes. Cut the rind from each slice, then cut the slices into smaller chunks.
2. In a blender, combine the cantaloupe with the yogurt, ginger, lime juice, honey, mint, basil, and salt and purée until smooth. (You may need to add a few tablespoons of water to reach the desired consistency.) Serve cold, in pretty little bowls. A little extra

chopped basil or mint sprinkled on top will add the perfect touch.

Note: A cantaloupe is ripe when it's pinkish-yellow rather than green and you can smell a fruity odor at the stem end.

Summer Cantaloupe Salad

Special equipment: none
Preparation: 5 minutes
Cooking: none
Servings: 4 adults or older children

Now that you've incorporated cantaloupe into your daily routine (or even if you haven't), try branching out! The acidity of the tomatoes and lime (and raspberries, if using) make this salad shine. Bonus: blend leftovers together and freeze to make a granita (see page 307).

Kids love to make this salad!

1 small ripe cantaloupe
180g cherry tomatoes, halved
2 tablespoons chopped fresh mint leaves
Juice of 1 lime (2 tablespoons) or ½ lemon (1 tablespoon)
⅛ teaspoon ground ginger, optional (see Note)
60g raspberries, for garnish, optional

1. Using a sharp knife, cut the melon in half and, using a spoon, scoop out the seeds (discard seeds). Slice each half lengthwise to make "smile" (crescent) shapes. Cut the rind from each slice, then cut the slices into smaller chunks.

2. In a large bowl, combine the cantaloupe, tomatoes, mint, lime juice, and ginger, if using, and toss lightly to combine. Garnish with raspberries, if desired.

Note: If you use the ginger, whisk it into the lime juice first, before adding it to the salad.

CITRUS

B TANGY CITRUS
SMOOTHIE

WE LOVE
SOUR!

C ORANGE OLIVE OIL
CAKE

D ZESTY ORANGE SALAD

Tangy Citrus Smoothie

Special equipment: blender
Preparation: 4 minutes
Cooking: none
Servings: 2 adults and 2 children (small "tasting" servings)

Smoothies (just like soups) are a great way to introduce new flavors to your kids. The creamy, smooth texture makes them a natural hit with kids of all ages. Plus, they're versatile: my test families served this recipe for breakfast, snack, and dessert!

Note: I wouldn't recommend serving this before a child is 12 months old, and then only in small quantities (and test these ingredients, one by one, with your child first to watch for any allergic reactions). If they do react, best to wait. My older daughter used to react to tomatoes (a red rash around the mouth), and my younger one to kiwis. This eventually went away by itself. No rush! This recipe is very flexible, so you can mix and match ingredients. Kids love experimenting in the kitchen, and coming up with "their" smoothie recipe is a lot of fun (and a great way to get them taste testing!).

By the way, if you don't like smoothies, this recipe might change your mind. My test families report that those who don't like the standard smoothie flavors (such as berry) were surprised to find the citrus to be so tasty!

240ml orange juice
Juice of ½ lemon (about 1 tablespoon)
1 big ripe banana or 2 small
120ml plain yogurt
One of the following: half a peeled grapefruit, 1 peeled kiwi, or 200g diced pineapple

2 ice cubes
2 tablespoons liquid honey
1 ripe avocado, pitted and peeled, optional

1. In a blender, combine the orange juice, lemon juice, banana, yogurt (use flavored if your kids are not yet citrus lovers), your choice of fruit, ice cubes, honey, and avocado, if using (also a good idea if your kids are not yet citrus lovers), and blend until smooth and frothy.

Taste-Training Tips:
Smoothies concentrate flavors, making them more intense. For younger kids or those new to tangy tastes, this smoothie will probably need the yogurt as well as the avocado, which will reduce the acidity level and balance the sour taste, making it interesting rather than overly strong.

I serve this recipe in tiny kid-size teacups or tall, thin juice glasses (or even cocktail glasses). This is a "tasting" recipe, so kids don't need a lot.

Orange Olive Oil Cake

Special equipment: 20- or 23-cm round cake pan; electric mixer
Preparation: 10 minutes
Cooking: 30 minutes
Servings: 8 slices

This is not a new idea, but that doesn't make it any less worth including! This is one of my favorite cake recipes of all time. Tangy yet sweet, the flavors are best when this cake has been allowed to sit for a day.

2 large eggs
150g granulated sugar
120ml olive oil
1 tablespoon orange zest
Juice of 1 orange (about 120ml)
30g poppy seeds, optional
215g plain flour, plus more for dusting
1 tablespoon baking powder
¼ teaspoon sea salt
Confectioner's (icing) sugar, for sprinkling

1. Preheat the oven to 180°C/gas 4. Grease and flour the cake pan.
2. In a large bowl, using an electric mixer on medium-high speed, mix the eggs and sugar until pale and fluffy, 3 to 4 minutes. With the mixer on, gradually add the olive oil in a thin stream, mixing until fluffy and light. Add the orange zest, orange juice, and poppy seeds, if using, and mix until well combined.
3. In a medium bowl, combine the flour, baking powder, and salt. With the mixer on low speed, add half the dry ingredients to the wet ingredients, mix until combined, then add the remaining dry ingredients and mix until just combined (don't overmix!).
4. Pour the batter into the prepared cake pan and bake for 30 minutes, or until the top springs back when touched. Remove the pan from the oven, allow to cool slightly, then turn out onto a wire rack and set aside to cool completely. To serve, sprinkle with confectioner's sugar and cut into wedges. This cake stores beautifully for up to a week in the fridge or for a few days stored in an airtight container at room temperature.

Taste-Training Tip: For kids who are cautious about citrus, make this with the orange juice only, then gradually introduce more and more orange zest. The cake will be tangier (but not sour). This is a great way to introduce them to bitter tastes.

> *This was super easy to make! My 6-year-old daughter loved it. First she said, "Deeeeliciouuuus" then, "Buttery and salty and sweet, and I like the crust part the best."*
> —Analis

Zesty Orange Salad

Special equipment: none
Preparation: 5 minutes
Cooking: 10 minutes
Servings: 2 adults and 2 children

This is one of the recipes in *French Kids Eat Everything*, and I couldn't resist introducing it again here. It's a dessert salad, which is a great way to introduce new flavors to children. The sweetness of the orange offsets the bitterness of the orange zest. Children will be reassured by the familiar (the pieces of orange) and so hopefully will be more willing to try something new (the thin, almost playful curlicues of sweetened orange rind).

Have your children watch you prepare this dish and let them try a sample if they're curious. When serving, remember that eating can sometimes be about encountering new tastes rather than consuming large quantities.

Serve this dish in a quiet moment when you have the time to sit and discuss the ingredients with your child. Questions are usually helpful (and helpfully distracting): How does the orange zest taste? Does it taste orangey at all? How does it taste when you nibble a tiny bit? Place a tiny piece on your tongue? What does it smell like? If your child doesn't want to eat any, that's fine, too, but encourage them to taste it.

Our daughters graduated from this to eating grapefruit, which they now enjoy as a breakfast treat. Claire, our younger daughter, will purse her lips and say, "Ooohhh, *Maman, c'est amer!* (it's bitter!)," and then continue eating with delight.

Because of its sweetness, the French would serve this as a dessert, even though it's called a salad.

4 seedless oranges
4 tablespoons granulated sugar

1. Wash 1 orange, dry it, and use a zester to peel all of the yummy zest. (If you don't have a zester, use a sharp paring knife to carefully peel the outer layer, taking only the very outside of the rind and avoiding the white pith underneath. Slice the zest into very thin strips. Extra points for making curlicues by slicing around the orange!)

2. Make the syrup: In a small saucepan over low heat, combine 120ml of water and the sugar and cook for 5 minutes, stirring often, until the sugar is completely dissolved. Add the zest and simmer for 10 minutes, or until the zest is tender (the syrup may start to turn a golden color, which is fine).

3. Meanwhile, peel the remaining oranges, completely cutting off and discarding any zest and pith so that you are left with just the fruit itself. Slice the oranges crosswise into thin circles and divide them evenly among 4 small salad bowls. Pour the zest and syrup over the top. Serve immediately!

PEACHES

A PEACHES & CREAM
PUREE

B LOVELY MINT LEMONADE

C 'MAGIC SPICE'
POACHED PEACHES

D SAVORY PEACH SALAD

Peaches and Cream Purée

Special equipment: blender
Preparation: 2 minutes
Cooking: 2 minutes
Servings: 3 or 4 baby jars

Baby fruit purées tend to get a little repetitive. Using peaches as your base is a great way to introduce little palates to the taste of a slightly more acidic fruit. Peaches and cream is a wonderful taste combination for adults, and this recipe follows the same flavor principle for baby!

1 ripe peach, peeled and quartered
1 teaspoon reduced-fat cream or whipping cream or 1 tablespoon plain Greek yogurt
⅛ teaspoon ground cinnamon

1. In a saucepan over high heat, bring 480ml of water to a boil. Once boiling, add the peach and cook for about 2 minutes, or until tender. Remove the pan from the heat and strain the peach, reserving the cooking liquid. (It will already smell wonderful by now.)
2. In a blender, combine the cooked peach, cream, and cinnamon and purée until smooth, adding enough cooking liquid to reach a desired consistency. Enjoy!

Taste-Training Tip: For older babies, try varying the flavor. In place of the cinnamon, add ⅛ teaspoon ground ginger, 1 teaspoon lemon or orange juice, ¼ teaspoon dried mint, or just the tiniest bit of pure vanilla extract.

Adult Serving Tip: This purée makes a great sauce to serve with vanilla ice cream. Make 1 batch of the recipe for every two people and blend away! Garnish with fresh mint leaves—mint and peach are a nice flavor combination.

Lovely Peachy Mint Lemonade

Special equipment: citrus juicer; large pitcher
Preparation: 5 minutes
Cooking: 10 minutes
Servings: 480 to 720ml

Even humble lemonade can act as a vehicle for new and fun tastes. Who would have thought this taste combination would work? But it does, to perfection. (Confession: I sometimes make this using store-bought lemonade. If you don't feel like squeezing all of those lemons, it's an option!)

2 peaches, pitted, peeled, and chopped
50g granulated sugar
30g chopped fresh mint leaves
Juice of 8 lemons (about 240ml)
½ lemon, thinly sliced, for garnish
15g whole mint leaves, for garnish

1. In a small saucepan over high heat, combine the peaches, sugar, chopped mint leaves, and 240ml of water and bring to a boil, stirring constantly. When the sugar has dissolved, after about 2 minutes, reduce the heat to medium-low and simmer for 5 more minutes. Remove the pan from the heat and set aside to cool, then transfer the syrup to an airtight container and refrigerate (see Note).

2. Using a fine-mesh sieve set over a pitcher half-filled with ice cubes, strain the syrup (discard the solids). Add 480ml of water (or more as desired) and the lemon juice. Serve garnished with the lemon slices and whole mint leaves.

Note: This simple peach-mint syrup is best when made in advance and chilled. It will keep for up to 2 weeks in the fridge.

Adventurous Eating Tip: Try substituting basil for the mint— trust me, it's tasty!

"Magic Spice" Poached Peaches

Special equipment: none
Preparation: 5 minutes
Cooking: 20 minutes
Servings: 4 adults or older children

Poached fruit is one of our family's favorite desserts. Sure, there are more elegant ways to serve peaches, but this is a fast dessert to make, can be served hot or cold, and, when properly garnished, looks rather elegant, too! My younger daughter, Claire, calls this the "magic spice" recipe because of the star anise. And she's right: star anise does look a little magical (at least to a 4-year-old in "fairy mode"). The bonus: you can use frozen peaches. We buy fresh peaches when they're selling them by the case at the end of the summer, halve them, remove the stones, peel them, and freeze them in freezer bags. This way, we can poach them directly from the freezer. You can also buy frozen peaches at the grocery store.

115g dark brown sugar
One 5- to 8-cm cinnamon stick or 1 teaspoon ground cinnamon
3 whole star anise
5-mm piece fresh gingerroot, peeled and thinly sliced or 1 teaspoon ground ginger
4 ripe peaches, quartered
60g slivered almonds, optional

1. In a medium saucepan, combine the brown sugar, cinnamon, star anise, and ginger with 720ml of water. Bring to a boil over high heat, stirring often. Reduce the heat to medium-low and simmer, stirring occasionally, for about 10 minutes (the mixture will darken, and the flavors will slowly infuse the liquid). Add the peaches in a single layer. Cover, and simmer for 5 minutes. Using a spoon, gently turn the peaches over, cover, and simmer for another 5 minutes, or until tender. Remove the pan from the heat, leaving the peaches in the syrup and the lid firmly on to prevent the syrup from getting too thick, and set aside for 10 minutes. (The heat will gradually cook the peaches, but they'll stay firm.)

2. Meanwhile, in a small, dry frying pan over medium-high heat, toast the almond slivers until golden, 3 to 4 minutes (stir them often to avoid burning).

3. There are many ways to serve this dish. Try drizzling the cooked peaches with cream or spooning them over ice cream. Garnish with the toasted almonds. (If you add raspberry syrup and serve the peaches with ice cream, you'll be recreating the famous French dessert Peach Melba, which renowned chef Auguste Escoffier created in honor of the Australian soprano singer Nellie Melba. *Ooh la la!*)

Savory Peach Salad

Special equipment: none
Preparation: 5 minutes
Cooking: none
Servings: 4 adults or older children

I know, I know. You're probably thinking, *Rocket, for my kids?*
Are you kidding? Well, trust me and try this recipe. Italian kids
grow up eating this stuff. If you introduce rocket early enough,
they'll take to it like ducks to water. To get started, take a gradual approach. If your kids are enjoying peaches, then try
including just a little spinach. Then add a little rocket. Add whatever nuts they like (almonds? pistachios?). If they'll let you, add
a little goat cheese (or feta or blue cheese). Call it the "gradual
gourmet" method.

170g fresh raspberries
1 batch Classic Vinaigrette (page 365; see Note)
Sea salt and ground black pepper, optional
1 large or 2 small bunches baby spinach (about 300g)
4 large peaches, pitted and cut into bite-size pieces
40g sliced almonds, pistachios, or walnuts
1 small bag rocket
40g crumbled feta, goat, or blue cheese, optional

1. Make the vinaigrette: Press one third of the raspberries through a fine-mesh sieve set over a small bowl
   (discard the solids). Add the Classic Vinaigrette and
   whisk to combine. Taste and season with salt and
   pepper, if desired.
2. Make the salad: In a large salad bowl, gently toss 2
   to 3 tablespoons of the prepared vinaigrette with the

Fun with Flavors! Fruit Recipes 331

spinach, peaches, almonds, rocket, and cheese, if using (take care not to bruise the peaches). Reserve the rest of the vinaigrette to be added, as desired, on individual servings. (Kids often don't like salads that are overdressed—too "slimy"!). Garnish the salad with the remaining raspberries.

Note: If time is short (when isn't it?), use store-bought raspberry vinaigrette. Your kids will love it either way!

PEARS

 A PEAR-PLUM COMPOTE

B PLAYFUL PINK PEARS

C PLEASANT PEAR SOUP

D POIRES BELLE HELENE

Pear-Plum Compote

Special equipment: blender
Preparation: 3 minutes
Cooking: 5 minutes
Servings: 6 to 8 baby jars

On its own, pear compote can be slightly grainy, depending on the variety and ripeness of the pears. Combining pear with plum makes this compote smoother and just slightly more tangy—a nice contrast to the puréed apples and bananas your baby may already love.

1 ripe pear, peeled, quartered, and cored
1 large or 2 small ripe plums, peeled, quartered and pitted
⅛ teaspoon ground cinnamon

1. In a saucepan over high heat, bring 480ml of water to a boil and then add the pear and plums. Reduce the heat to medium-high and simmer until very tender, about 5 minutes. Remove the pan from the heat and strain the fruit, reserving the cooking liquid.
2. In a blender, combine the cooked fruit, cinnamon, and 120ml of the cooking liquid and purée until smooth. If needed, add more cooking liquid to reach the desired consistency.

Playful Pink Pears

Special equipment: none
Preparation: 5 minutes
Cooking: 20 minutes
Servings: 4 adults or older children

The flavor of pears really emerges when they're teamed with something slightly acidic. In this recipe, the cranberry juice does the trick. Plus it turns the pears bright pink, which creates a funny yet familiar dessert that will get your kids thinking about flavors.

720ml cranberry juice (see Note)
Liquid honey or stevia, to taste
2 whole star anise
One 5- to 7-cm cinnamon stick or 1 teaspoon ground cinnamon
2 whole cloves
4 ripe pears, quartered and cored

1. In a medium saucepan over high heat, bring the juice, honey, star anise, cinnamon, and cloves to a boil, stirring well. Reduce the heat to medium-low and simmer for about 10 minutes, stirring occasionally. Add the pears in a single layer, cover, and simmer for about 5 minutes. Gently turn the pears over, and simmer for 5 more minutes, or until just tender. Remove the pan from the heat, leaving the pears in the syrup and the lid firmly on the pan to prevent the syrup from becoming too thick. (The heat will gradually cook the pears, but they'll stay firm.) Set aside until cool, then transfer the pan to the fridge to chill the pears completely. Serve the pears cold with the syrup.

Note: If desired, you can use cranberry cocktail instead of cranberry juice; just omit the honey or stevia.

Taste-Training Tip: As you're eating, ask your children to guess how the pears turned pink. For older children, you can have them compare the flavor with cranberry juice, cranberry sauce, or (best of all) frozen raw cranberries. Can they taste the cranberry flavor in the pears?

Pleasant Pear Soup

Special equipment: blender
Preparation: 15 minutes
Cooking: 15 minutes
Servings: 4 servings (adults or older children)

For years, I avoided fennel in the grocery store. *What, exactly,* I wondered, *am I supposed to do with it?* I just assumed my kids wouldn't eat it. As with so many foods, I was delighted to be proven wrong—it's now a Le Billon family favorite. The fennel has a slight anise or licorice taste to it, which makes this soup sweet but interesting.

1 tablespoon salted butter
2 tablespoons olive oil
2 large or 3 small fennel bulbs, fronds removed, halved, cored, and cut into chunks
1 medium onion, thinly sliced
1 teaspoon sea salt
½ teaspoon ground black pepper
4 medium pears, peeled, cored, and quartered
2 potatoes, peeled and diced
240ml apple juice

1 litre *Brodo* (page 364) or ready-to-use low-sodium vegetable stock
1 bay leaf

1. In a large saucepan over medium-high heat, melt the butter in the oil. Add the fennel, onion, salt, and pepper. Reduce the heat to medium, cover, and cook, stirring often, until the onion begins to turn golden brown, 5 or 6 minutes. Add the pears and potatoes, increase the heat to high, and cook for 2 to 3 minutes. Reduce the heat to medium, add the apple juice, *brodo,* and bay leaf, cover, and simmer, stirring often, until the fennel, pears, and potatoes are tender, about 5 minutes. Remove the pan from the heat and discard the bay leaf.
2. Using a blender, purée the soup until smooth. Serve immediately.

Adventurous Eaters Tip: Garnish with freshly toasted fennel seeds for a crunchy, flavorful option.

Poires Belle Hélène (Beautiful Helen's Pears)

Special equipment: baking dish
Preparation: 30 minutes
Cooking: 15 minutes
Servings: 4 adults or older children

This amazing dessert is slightly out of fashion in France. It was invented in the 19th century and named after an opera about Helen of Troy by Jacques Offenbach. My husband ate it a lot growing up, when it was one of the most popular desserts at dinner parties. Other desserts are more popular among the

French these days so it took me a few years in France before I discovered this dish. When I did, I was immediately hooked.

The poached pears are drizzled with chocolate syrup (and, in some recipes, crystallized violets). Simpler versions (like this one) use sliced almonds instead of the violets. The combination of sweet pear with dark chocolate is irresistible. Plus, it feels incredibly indulgent while still being pretty healthy. American or British versions often add cream-based sauces, but this version is faithful to the French original, which is deceptively simple. *Bon appétit!*

4 ripe pears, peeled with the stems left on (see Notes)
1 tablespoon salted butter
115g dark or milk chocolate, chopped
120ml reduced-fat cream, whole milk, or milk alternative
1 teaspoon pure vanilla extract
60ml pure maple syrup
50g flaked or slivered almonds, optional (see Notes)

1. Make the poached pears: Using a paring knife, slice a thin layer off the bottom of each pear so that it can sit upright. Arrange the pears (upright) in a large saucepan and add enough water just to cover them. Remove the pears and set aside. Bring the water to a boil over high heat, gently lower each pear into the pan, and poach until the pears are tender when pierced with the point of a sharp knife, 10 to 12 minutes. (Don't undercook the pears: the goal is to have very tender pears that you can easily eat with a dessert spoon.) Using tongs, gently transfer the pears to a baking dish, discarding the poaching liquid. Cover and refrigerate to cool completely.

2. Make the chocolate sauce: In a small saucepan over low heat, melt the butter. Add the chocolate, cream and vanilla extract, and cook, stirring constantly, until the chocolate has completely melted. (Add a little extra

cream if the mixture seems too thick—it should be pourable.) Remove the pan from the heat and set aside to cool slightly. (If the sauce becomes too thick, you can thin it by stirring in 1 teaspoon of water at a time.)

3. When the pears are cooled, core them using an apple corer or your knife, working from the bottom to remove the seeds and leaving the stem intact. Set each cored pear upright in its own serving dish, drizzle with maple syrup, then with the chocolate sauce, adding enough so that each pear floats in its own little chocolate lake. Garnish with almonds, if using, and serve.

Notes: For this recipe, choose a variety of pear that holds up well when heated, such as Bosc pears. For an added touch, toast the almonds in a dry frying pan over low heat, stirring often, for 4 to 5 minutes or until just beginning to turn golden brown.

Taste-Training Tip: Once you have served this dessert once, experiment by adding new spices to the chocolate sauce. Ground cinnamon and ginger are popular options, or try orange zest. This is a great way to get your kids trying new flavor combinations. Why not let them take turns picking flavors and seeing how they turn out? Some families eat this with the maple syrup and nuts only—if you aren't chocolate fans, give it a try!

Great recipe, especially as we are trying to transition from having a sweet dessert every night to having fruit instead.

—Mira

STRAWBERRIES

STRAWBERRY RHUBARB
SAUCE

STRAWBERRY ALMOND
CLAFOUTIS

STRAWBERRY SPINACH
SALAD

Strawberry Rhubarb Sauce

Special equipment: blender
Preparation: 5 minutes
Cooking: 10 minutes
Servings: 4 adults or children

This is an exciting, fun purée that doubles as a great sauce for pouring over pancakes or splashing over ice cream. Or spooning over morning oatmeal. Or drizzling over yogurt. Did I mention I like this sauce?

This recipe freezes well, so I make a large batch in early summer, when the strawberries and rhubarb are both ripe. In fact, I love this recipe so much that I started growing strawberries and rhubarb in our garden!

100g granulated sugar
280g chopped rhubarb stalks
280g hulled and sliced strawberries
1 ripe banana

1. In a medium saucepan over medium heat, bring 120ml of water to a boil. Add the sugar and rhubarb and simmer until the rhubarb just starts to become tender, 3 to 4 minutes. Add the strawberries and simmer, stirring occasionally, until tender, 5 to 7 minutes. Add the banana and, using a blender, purée the mixture, adding 1 teaspoon of water at a time to reach the desired consistency. (Alternatively, transfer to a blender and purée.) Serve warm or cold, on just about anything!

Strawberry Almond Clafoutis

Special equipment: 20-cm square baking dish; food processor
Preparation: 15 minutes
Cooking: 45 minutes
Servings: 6 to 8 adults or children

Clafoutis are the French answer to strawberry shortcake: unpre-
tentious and reliably delicious. The fluffy custard is easy to make.
The almonds are mouth-wateringly good served with strawberries. What are you waiting for?

60g salted butter
70g plain flour
60g slivered or whole blanched almonds
100g granulated sugar, plus 2 teaspoons for garnish, optional
1 tablespoon cornflour
Pinch sea salt
3 large eggs
180ml whole milk
530g strawberries, rinsed, hulled, and quartered, plus a few more
for garnish
60g slivered almonds, optional
60ml whipping cream, optional

1. Preheat the oven to 180°C/gas 4. Grease a baking
    dish.
2. In a saucepan over low heat, melt the butter. Remove
    the pan from the heat and set aside.
3. In a food processor, combine the flour and blanched
    almonds and pulse until the almonds are finely
    ground. Add the sugar, cornflour, and salt, and pulse

to combine. Add the eggs, one by one, pulsing after each to combine. Add the melted butter and milk and process just until the mixture forms a batter the consistency of heavy cream.

4. Spread the strawberries in a single layer in the prepared baking dish. Pour the batter gently over the top, taking care not to disturb the strawberries. Bake in the oven until puffy and set, about 40 minutes. Remove the pan from the oven and set aside to cool. Serve warm or cold straight from the dish. Garnish with a sprinkling of sugar or slivered almonds, top with fresh strawberries, drizzle with cream, or enjoy it plain.

Strawberry Spinach Salad

Special equipment: none
Preparation: 5 minutes
Cooking: none
Servings: 4 adults or children

For many kids, the secret to accepting new vegetables (even typically disliked ones) is combining them with a bit of sweetness and healthy fat. (The good news is that healthy fat helps us absorb nutrients, and the vitamin C in the strawberries helps us absorb the iron in the spinach.) Boiled spinach is no fun, but this salad is delicious. *Parfait!*

3 tablespoons extra virgin olive oil
1 tablespoon balsamic vinegar
1 teaspoon pure maple syrup
Pinch sea salt and ground black pepper
2 small bunches or 1 large bunch baby spinach

350g strawberries, rinsed, hulled, and cut into bite-size pieces
60g slivered almonds, toasted
60g red onion, finely sliced, optional

1. In a large salad bowl, whisk together the oil, vinegar, maple syrup, salt, and pepper. Add the spinach, strawberries, almonds, and onion, if using, and gently toss to combine. Serve immediately (or else the spinach will wilt). *Voilà!*

Taste-Training Tip: If you're not sure your kids will like this, go back a step. Introduce them to the taste of spinach using the recipes on pages 262 and 263. Or toss some strawberries with the vinaigrette one day, just to try. They'll get there!

WATERMELON

MELON LOVERS OF THE WORLD UNITE!

 B WATERMELON STARS

 C WATERMELON SOUP

  D WATERMELON, LIME, AND FETA SALAD

Watermelon Stars

Special equipment: star-shaped cookie cutter (or any other shape you like)
Preparation: 5 minutes
Cooking: none
Servings: as many as you like!

This simple, fun recipe is a great way to introduce toddlers to watermelon. They'll love helping you make the stars. (Warning: this usually gets messy!)

1 small seedless watermelon

1. Cut the watermelon into slices about 1-cm thick. Lay the slices flat on a cutting board or baking sheet. Using a cookie cutter(s), cut fun shapes from the watermelon (roundish shapes work best). (The leftovers make great juice—just blend, strain, and serve with a squeeze of lime juice! Will keep in the fridge for a day or two.)

Watermelon Soup

Special equipment: blender
Preparation: 10 minutes plus 3 hours for chilling
Cooking: none
Servings: 4 to 6 adults or older children

Maybe it's because I have two little girls, but I find pink foods super-appealing. This soup can be served as a summer soup all on its own or as a dessert soup any time of year.

½ small seedless watermelon, chopped
1 cucumber, peeled, seeded, and coarsely chopped
240ml plain Greek yogurt, plus extra for garnish
Juice from 2 lemons or 3 to 4 limes (about 4 tablespoons)
Pinch sea salt
15g chopped fresh mint leaves, for garnish
Liquid honey, for garnish

1. In a blender, combine the watermelon, cucumber, yogurt, lemon juice, and salt and purée until smooth. Transfer to an airtight container and chill for 3 hours (or overnight). To serve, ladle into bowls and garnish with mint and drizzles of yogurt and honey, if desired. (You may need to mix a bit of water into the yogurt for it to drizzle.)

Watermelon, Lime, and Feta Salad

Special equipment: none
Preparation: 7 minutes
Cooking: none
Serving: 4 to 6 adults or children

Most children love watermelon, so this is a great way to introduce them to feta cheese (which many young children adore, surprisingly). The three flavors of watermelon, lime, and feta remind me of southern France, where this is a traditional late-summer salad.

½ small seedless watermelon, chopped; see Note
150g crumbled feta cheese
30g minced fresh coriander leaves or minced fresh mint and basil leaves

10 black olives, pitted and chopped into small pieces, optional
Juice of 2 limes (about 2 tablespoons) or to taste

1. Arrange the watermelon in a single layer on a serving
    plate, sprinkle with feta, coriander, and olives, if
    using. (Do not toss!) Drizzle the lime juice over the
    entire plate and allow guests to serve themselves.

Note: Watermelon cuts easily with cookie cutters. Use them to
serve a whimsical version of this salad to your child (have them
help cut out the shapes!).

Baby's Birthday Yogurt Cake with Chocolate Avocado Icing

Special equipment: 23-cm round cake pan; parchment paper; food processor
Preparation: 20 minutes plus 10 minutes for cooling
Cooking: 35 minutes
Servings: 8 adults or children (small slices)

This (relatively) healthy yogurt cake is one of the most traditional French dessert recipes and is often one of the first desserts that French children make at home. It's easy to make (and relatively hard to ruin). We love to serve this as a birthday cake—it's *that* good.

Yogurt cake has a simple, moist texture that children love. The lemon zest and slightly tangy flavor from the yogurt offset the sweetness of the cake nicely. Perfect at any time of day.

I've added a very North American twist: avocado icing. (Not well known in France, I must say!) It was a hit with my test families and is a lovely, creamy alternative to butter.

The cake can be made in advance and stored, tightly covered, in the refrigerator for up to 2 days, but the icing is best made right before serving.

Yogurt Cake:
240ml plain Greek yogurt
140g granulated sugar
2 large eggs
80ml vegetable oil
1 teaspoon pure vanilla extract
1 tablespoon finely grated lemon zest
350g plain flour
1½ teaspoons baking powder
½ teaspoon bicarbonate of soda
¼ teaspoon sea salt

Chocolate Avocado Icing:
2 large avocados, pitted and peeled
1 teaspoon pure vanilla extract
2 tablespoons unsalted butter, softened, optional
140 to 280g confectioner's (icing) sugar
¼ teaspoon ground cinnamon
¼ teaspoon sea salt
6 tablespoons cocoa powder

1. Preheat the oven to 180°C/gas 4. Butter the cake pan and line the bottom with parchment paper.
2. In a large mixing bowl, whisk together the yogurt and sugar. Add the eggs one at a time, beating well after each addition. Add the vegetable oil, vanilla, and lemon zest and whisk to combine.
3. In a separate bowl, whisk together the flour, baking powder, bicarbonate of soda, and salt. Fold the dry ingredients into the wet ingredients until just combined. (Don't overmix!)
4. Pour the batter into the prepared cake pan and bake in the oven until golden brown on top or until a knife inserted into the middle of the cake comes out clean, about 30 to 35 minutes. Remove the pan from the oven and allow the cake to cool in the pan for 10

minutes, then turn out onto a wire rack to cool completely before icing.

5. Make the icing: In a food processor, combine the avocado, vanilla, and butter, if desired, and process until smooth. With the motor running, add the sugar a little bit at a time, followed by the cinnamon, salt, and cocoa powder. Add up to another 140g of sugar, to taste. If the icing is a little chunky, try gradually adding a little bit of cream until you achieve the right consistency.

6. Ice the cake: Transfer the cake to a serving platter. Using a spatula, place a large amount of icing on the center of the cake. Gently smooth out the icing toward the edges until the top is evenly covered. Cover the sides with icing. Smooth the sides by slowly spinning the plate while holding the spatula to the icing surface. Repeat with the remaining icing until the top and sides are evenly covered.

Taste-Training Tip: If you're really adventurous, frost your cake with gorgeously green Lemon-Avocado Icing instead. Follow the directions above, substituting 1 tablespoon lemon juice for the cocoa powder and adding at least an extra 70g confectioner's (icing) sugar to achieve the right consistency. For this version, serve the cake immediately after frosting—it tends to turn brown with time.

I made the Avocado Icing for my son's birthday. There were 10 kids present and not one of them blinked an eye at it. It looks—and tastes—exactly like regular chocolate icing!

—Roberta

Almond Mini-Cakes (*Financiers*)

B **C** **D**

Special equipment: mini-muffin pan
Preparation: 10 minutes plus at least 10 minutes for cooling
Cooking: 15 minutes
Servings: makes about 2 dozen

These little almond tea cakes are utterly irresistible. In their small, rectangular version, they are often served as an after-dinner *mignardise,* which comes from the old-fashioned French word *mignard* (a small child, particularly a graceful, sweet one). Sums it up perfectly!

Wonderful bonus: these are gluten-free, as they use almond flour instead of wheat flour. If you can't find almond flour, you can make your own by using your food processor to grind up blanched almonds. The consistency won't be as fine, but the cakes will still be yummy!

90g salted butter
90g almond flour
90g confectioner's (icing) sugar
4 tablespoons cocoa powder
⅛ teaspoon sea salt
2 large egg whites
¼ teaspoon pure almond extract

1. Preheat the oven to 180°C/gas 5. Lightly grease a mini-muffin pan.
2. In a small saucepan over low heat, melt the butter. Remove the pan from the heat and set it aside to cool (if the butter is too hot, it will cook the egg whites— disastrous!).
3. In a large mixing bowl, whisk together the flour,

sugar, cocoa powder, and salt. Stir in the egg whites and almond extract, then gradually stir in the cooled melted butter and mix until smooth.

4. Pour the batter into the mini-muffin pan, filling each cup about three-quarters full. Bake in the oven until the cakes are puffy and slightly springy to the touch, 12 to 15 minutes. Remove from the oven and set aside to cool completely (if you try to remove them from the molds while they're still warm they'll break!). The cakes will keep for up to a week stored in an airtight container at room temperature.

Adventurous Eater Tip: Substitute ½ teaspoon chopped culinary lavender for the almond extract.

No-Bake Choco-Raisin Treats (*Mendiants*)

Special equipment: silicon muffin cups or parchment paper
Preparation: 30 minutes plus about 30 minutes to set
Cooking: none
Servings: about 8 large cookies or 16 smaller cookies

These fun chocolate treats taste decadent but are (relatively) low in sugar—and they're a lighter alternative to filling chocolate cake. Who would have thought something this easy to make could be so delicious?

A *mendiant* (the traditional French word for this dessert) is a chocolate disk studded with nuts and dried fruits: raisins, hazelnuts, figs, and almonds. Traditionally eaten at Christmas, they're now eaten year round, and endless varieties can be found that incorporate everything from seeds to fruit peel. Use your imagination! The goal is to have your children enjoying making food and being in the kitchen, so try to make these together.

1 tablespoon unsalted butter
225g dark or milk chocolate, chopped
1 teaspoon ground cinnamon
1 tablespoon whipping cream (if you are using dark chocolate)
60g slivered or sliced almonds
60g dried blueberries

1. In a small saucepan over low heat, melt the butter. Add the chocolate and stir continuously, until completely melted. Add the cinnamon and, if using dark chocolate, cream.

2. Assemble the cookies: You can do this using either silicone muffin cups (my preference) or parchment paper. If using muffin cups, drop about 1 heaped tablespoon of the melted chocolate mixture into the bottom of three or four muffin cups at a time. If using parchment paper, lay the parchment on a flat work surface and drop small spoonfuls of chocolate on the sheet, about three or four at a time, using the back of the spoon to make little circles about 5 cm in diameter. Before the chocolate hardens, add the almonds and blueberries in any design you like—use your imagination! (If the chocolate mixture hardens before you have finished, don't worry: you can re-melt it.)

3. Set the cookies aside to harden, testing the edges cautiously until you are sure they are ready (at least 30 minutes). *Yum!*

Taste-Training Tip: I've suggested blueberries and almonds in this recipe, but start with toppings your children already love then introduce new flavors. Toppings can include nuts (almonds, pistachios, pralines, pecans), dried fruit (raisins, blueberries, thinly sliced apricots, cranberries, crystallized ginger or orange rind), or even fleur de sel, seeds, or chunks of your favorite cookies!

These were a hit with my boys (ages 6 and 4). They declared them the best cookies that I've ever made and had fun adding granola and fresh raspberries and strawberries as toppings.

—Stacy

Cinnamon and Clove Biscuits

Special equipment: baking sheet; parchment paper; cookie cutter
Preparation: 20 minutes
Cooking: 10 minutes
Servings: makes 2 dozen small biscuits

Teething babies love to gnaw on almost anything, but traditional baby biscuits are fairly plain. Why not spice it up? Clove oil is traditionally used to help soothe toothache, and this recipe uses a bit of ground clove to give the biscuits a unique taste.

85g dry infant oat cereal
215g plain flour or wheat flour or oat flour
1 teaspoon ground cinnamon
½ teaspoon ground cloves
6 tablespoons melted butter
2 very ripe bananas, mashed until smooth

1. Preheat the oven to 220°C/gas 7. Line a baking sheet with parchment paper.
2. In a large mixing bowl, whisk together the cereal, flour, cinnamon and cloves. Gradually stir in the butter, then mix in the banana. (The dough should be soft and smooth; if it is too dry, add 1 tablespoon of water at a time—how much you'll need will depend on how large and ripe the banana is.) Using your

hands, form the dough into a ball and then roll it out on a floured work surface to 6-mm thickness. Using a cookie cutter, cut into circles or ovals (no pointy edges or corners for baby!). Transfer the shapes to the prepared baking sheet and bake in the oven until lightly browned, 7 to 10 minutes. Remove from the oven and set aside to cool completely on the baking sheet before serving. The cookies will keep in an airtight container at room temperature for up to 1 week.

Safety Tip: As with any teething biscuit, watch your child closely to make sure the biscuit doesn't pose a choking hazard.

Lemon Mousse

Special equipment: none
Preparation: 10 minutes plus 2 hours for chilling
Cooking: 10 minutes
Servings: 4 adults or 8 children

When you mention the word "mousse," most people think of chocolate. But lemon mousse works wonderfully, too. With very little cream, this mousse is a light and airy, melt-in-your-mouth treat.

4 large eggs
200g granulated sugar
¼ teaspoon sea salt
Zest of 2 lemons (about 1 heaped tablespoon)
Juice of 2 lemons (about 4 tablespoons)
120ml whipping cream
½ teaspoon pure vanilla extract
Garnish: very thin lemon slices, fresh berries, or fresh mint leaves

1. Make the lemon curd: In two small bowls, separate the egg yolks from the whites, setting the whites aside for later.

2. In a cool, medium saucepan, whisk together the egg yolks and half the sugar, then whisk in the salt and lemon zest and juice until smooth. Cook the mixture over medium heat, stirring often, until thickened to the consistency of a not-quite-set pudding, about 10 minutes. Pour the mixture through a fine-mesh sieve into a large bowl (discard any solids). Cover with plastic wrap and chill in the fridge until firm (at least 1 hour, more if possible).

3. Make the mousse: In a bowl, whisk together the egg whites and the remaining sugar until stiff peaks form, then gently fold in the chilled lemon curd. In another bowl, whisk together the cream and vanilla until stiff peaks form. Fold the whipped cream into the lemon mixture until just combined (don't over-stir!).

4. Spoon the mousse into little individual serving ramekins or cups and chill for at least 1 hour, or until firm to the touch. Serve with your choice of garnish.

Safety Tip: This dish does include raw egg whites, which according to medical advice in some countries should not be given to babies under 12 months.

Roast Pineapple Surprise

Special equipment: baking sheet; parchment paper; aluminum foil
Preparation: 5 minutes
Cooking: 15 minutes

Servings: 8 children or 4 adults (depending on the size of your pineapple)

This simple yet delicious dessert is really quick. Prepare the pineapple as your dinner is cooking, then let it bake while you're eating. It's a classic French approach: lots of fruit, a little sugar, and an intriguing flavor twist.

1 ripe pineapple
60g dark brown sugar
½ teaspoon ground ginger
½ teaspoon ground cinnamon
½ teaspoon ground allspice
Juice of ½ lemon (about 1 tablespoon)
Vanilla or coconut ice cream or gelato, for serving

1. Preheat the oven to 160°C/gas 3. Line a baking sheet with parchment paper.
2. Remove the pineapple's spiky leaves by twisting them away from the crown. Core the pineapple. Using a sharp knife, cut the unpeeled pineapple into slices approximately 2.5-cm thick. Arrange the slices in a single layer, flesh-side up, on the prepared baking sheet.
3. In a small bowl, combine the brown sugar, ginger, cinnamon, allspice, lemon juice, and 60ml of water. Drizzle the mixture over the pineapple slices. Cover tightly with aluminum foil. Bake in the oven for about 15 minutes, or until tender, basting once or twice with the juice in the pan. Serve with ice cream. *Yum!*

Lemon Ginger Thyme Shortbread

Ⓑ   Ⓒ   Ⓓ

Special equipment: mixer; baking sheet; parchment paper; pastry brush
Preparation: 15 minutes plus 1 hour for chilling
Cooking: 15 minutes
Servings: makes at least 2 dozen cookies

Shortbread is a perennial kids' favorite. This recipe spices it up with a bit of ginger and thyme. Sounds odd, I know, but trust me: this is a really delicious combination!

645g plain flour
¼ teaspoon sea salt
2 teaspoons baking powder
1 teaspoon dried thyme
225g unsalted butter, at room temperature
200g granulated sugar
2 tablespoons lemon zest
1 teaspoon ground ginger
1 large egg
Juice of 1 lemon (about 2 tablespoons)
60ml whole milk

1. Preheat the oven to 160°C/gas 3. Line a baking sheet with parchment paper.
2. In a large bowl, combine the flour, salt, baking powder, and thyme. Set aside.
3. Using a mixer on medium-high speed, cream the butter, sugar, lemon zest, and ginger until fluffy, 3 to 5 minutes. Add the egg and lemon juice and mix on medium speed until combined. Add the flour mixture and mix on low speed just until incorporated (don't

overmix). Divide the dough in half and, using your hands, shape each piece into a log (they'll be about 7.5-cm thick). Wrap in plastic wrap and chill in the fridge for at least 1 hour (or freeze for 15 minutes).

4. Unwrap the dough and cut the logs into 1.5-cm-thick slices. Arrange the cookies 2.5 cm apart on the prepared baking sheet. Using a pastry brush, brush the cookies with milk. Bake in the oven for 12 to 15 minutes, or until the edges turn golden. *Yum!*

Warm Chocolate Ginger Fondant Cake

This dessert has a soft center that oozes out of the cake when you cut it. That's why these are baked in little muffin cups or ramekins—so everyone can enjoy the ooze at their own pace. The most important step in this recipe is buttering the muffin cups really, really well so that the mini-cakes can slide out without breaking.

Special equipment: muffin pan or ramekins; paper muffin liners; baking sheet (optional)
Preparation: 20 minutes plus 1 hour for chilling
Cooking: 15 minutes
Servings: about 1 dozen small cakes

150g salted butter
115g dark chocolate, chopped into 1.5-cm pieces
130g granulated sugar
4 large eggs
100g plain flour
1 teaspoon ground ginger
Vanilla ice cream, for serving

1. Grease 2 x 6 muffin cups, line with paper muffin liners, then butter the muffin liners (important!).
2. In a small saucepan over low heat, combine the butter and chocolate and gently stir until completely melted.
3. Meanwhile, in a large mixing bowl, combine the sugar and eggs and beat until the mixture is pale, thick, and just starting to stick together (pastry chefs refer to this as a "ribbony" texture, because when you lift your mixing spoon the batter pours back into the bowl in thick ribbons).
4. In a separate bowl, mix the flour and ginger until well combined. Stir the flour into the egg mixture until combined, then add the chocolate mixture, stirring until smooth. Pour the batter into the (well-greased!) muffin cups, then cover with plastic wrap and chill for at least 30 minutes or, preferably, 1 hour. (If you're using ramekins, I suggest arranging them on a baking sheet before you pop them in the fridge.)
5. When you are nearly ready to serve, preheat the oven to 200°C/gas 6. Bake until the top of each cake is set, 12 to 13 minutes. Remove the muffin cups from the oven and set aside for at least 5 minutes to cool. Serve warm or with a little vanilla ice cream, if desired.

Taste-Training Tip: Experiment with this recipe to vary the flavour: try adding 1 teaspoon pure vanilla extract or ½ teaspoon pure almond, orange, or lavender extract. Or try adding 1 teaspoon ground cinnamon or substituting 1 teaspoon dried mint for the ground ginger. Make a game out of asking your kids to guess which flavor you've added.

Cat's Tongue Cookies (*Langues-de-Chat*)

B **C** **D**

Special equipment: baking sheet; parchment paper; mixer
Preparation: 10 minutes
Cooking: 7 minutes
Servings: at least 2 dozen cookies

These easy-to-make cookies are literally melt-in-your-mouth delicious. Experts will tell you to use a piping bag to get precise shapes, but for kids, I simply recommend that you let them spread the batter on their own to create lots of fun shapes.

115g unsalted butter
70g confectioner's (icing) sugar
3 large egg whites
½ teaspoon pure vanilla extract
215g plain flour
¼ teaspoon sea salt
Zest of 1 lemon

1. Preheat the oven to 190°C/gas 5. Line a baking sheet with parchment paper, then generously grease it with butter. (Trust me, do not put these cookies on the baking sheet directly, even if it is well-greased: they will likely break when you try to remove them.)
2. In a mixer on high speed, cream the butter until smooth. Add the sugar and beat until fluffy. Beat in the egg whites, then add the vanilla and mix until incorporated. Using a wooden spoon, gently fold in the flour and salt, scraping down the sides of the bowl as needed, then stir in the lemon zest.
3. Using the back of a spoon, spread the batter onto the baking sheet in "cat's tongue" shapes (roughly

oval), then bake in the oven until the cookies start
to turn golden at the edges, 5 to 7 minutes. Remove
the baking sheet from the oven and immediately
slide the cookies onto a wire rack to cool (if you
let them cool on the baking sheet, they'll be more
likely to break when you remove them—do it
while they're still warm!). Cool completely before
serving.

Taste-Training Tip: Try serving these cookies alongside other
desserts, such as the Lemon Mousse (page 355) or Verrines
(below) to add a little texture contrast.

Verrines (The No Fuss, No Muss, Elegant Dessert-in-a-Glass)

Special equipment: narrow glasses
Preparation: 10 minutes
Cooking: none
Servings: 6 to 12 (depending on the size and shape of your glasses)

Verrines are a standby in France, served for apéritifs (when you'd
be likely to find layers of savory ingredients like avocado and
crab mousse) or dessert. The way they are served says a lot
about the French approach to food: it needs to be a feast for the
eyes as well as the stomach. Your verrine will look a lot like a
parfait, and you'll serve it with a spoon. The kids will be intrigued
by the layers and will soon be asking to make their own. I've
suggested a basic recipe below, but the standard method is to
alternate dairy and fruit layers. Be creative—the possibilities are
endless!

Choose clear, narrow glasses for serving. A small juice glass might work well, or even a wine glass, but forgo the traditional sundae-size container—this is a "less is more" dessert.

1 recipe Berry Compote (page 333)
240ml plain Greek yogurt
140g fresh blueberries and raspberries, for garnish

1. In each glass, carefully spoon about 4 tablespoons Pear Plum Compote. Using a clean spoon, carefully top each with about 4 tablespoons yogurt, creating a clean second layer. Repeat until you have the desired number of beautiful layers. Garnish with blueberries and raspberries. Serve immediately or refrigerate and serve within a few hours.

Friendly Flavors: Basic Recipes

These quick and easy make-at-home basics give you four options for using familiar flavors to introduce new foods to your children. These recipes will also save you money while introducing your child to salt- and sugar-free variations on store-bought items. *Brodo*, for example, is a homemade vegetable stock that is a tasty base for baby purées as well as adult soups. Classic Vinaigrette is a tangy, healthy alternative to store-bought salad dressing. The Quick Crunchy Casserole features a yummy, crunchy texture that will help you introduce new veggies in a delicious, reassuring way. And the *Pistou* (a.k.a. "green ketchup") is a tasty and healthy alternative to that good ol' red stuff.

Brodo (Vegetable Stock)

Special equipment: none
Preparation: 5 minutes
Cooking: 30 minutes
Servings: makes about 500ml

Brodo is the Italian word for "broth," which is precisely the right way to describe this vegetable soup: subtle and tasty. Italian parents make this stock in batches and either freeze or refrigerate it. At first, they serve it on its own, but it quickly becomes the basis for other soups and purées. Italians are told by their pediatricians to mix it with rice cereal and to add a dollop of olive oil and a sprinkle of grated Parmesan (Parmigiano-Reggiano) before serving. This results in a melt-in-your-mouth *pappa* that Italian babies love.

1 medium potato, peeled and cut into 2.5-cm cubes
1 large carrot, peeled and chopped
1 large zucchini, chopped
1 small baby leek, white part only, thinly sliced, optional

1. In a large saucepan over medium heat, simmer the potato, carrot, zucchini, and leek in 1 litre of water until the liquid is reduced by half, about 30 minutes (as the mixture simmers, it will thicken). Strain the soup through a fine-mesh sieve (discard solids) and set aside to cool.

Note: This recipe can easily be doubled. *Brodo* will keep in the fridge (tightly covered) for 2 to 3 days and in the freezer for up to a month.

Friendly Flavor Tip: Use *Brodo* as a base for your baby purées or soups. It will lend a rich underlying flavor that kids will find reassuringly familiar, which will help them get acquainted faster with new foods and tastes as you vary the purée/soup recipes.

Classic Vinaigrette

Special equipment: resealable glass jar
Preparation: 2 to 3 minutes
Cooking: none
Makes: about 200ml

This vinaigrette is incredibly versatile. Serve it as a salad dressing or as a dip for vegetables. Before the main evening meal, for example, I serve the vinaigrette in little individual bowls along with crudités (raw vegetables) such as carrots and cucumber sticks. For a snack, sometimes my daughters prepare veggie trays in mini-muffin tins, filling each hole with different veggies and one hole with vinaigrette. Kids like cute things and fun presentation!

The vinaigrette will keep in an airtight container in the fridge for up to 1 week. It saves money and is healthier, too!

120ml extra virgin olive oil or other high-quality vegetable oil
60ml vinegar
½ tablespoon Dijon-style mustard
1 tablespoon pure maple syrup, optional
1 tablespoon finely minced shallot, scallion, or onion, optional

1. In a resealable glass jar, combine the oil, vinegar, mustard, maple syrup, and shallot and shake vigorously. Taste before serving and adjust the seasonings to your preference (my mother-in-law prefers a more acidic vinaigrette, whereas I prefer a slightly sweeter, gentler version).

Taste-Training Tip: Kids love using the vinaigrette as a dip (my younger daughter would eat it with a spoon if I let her!). Once they are familiar with this flavor, encourage your child to try new veggies by dipping them in the vinaigrette.

Quick Crunchy Casserole

Special equipment: 20- x 25-cm baking dish
Preparation: 15 minutes
Cooking: 10 minutes
Servings: 4 adults and older children

This casserole is based on the French gratin cooking technique, used to serve a variety of vegetables from potatoes to cauliflower. *Gratin* refers to a white sauce and crunchy topping that lends savory flavor to vegetables. Once kids are used to gratin-style dishes, this is a wonderful way to get them to try new foods: the gratin sauce and topping provides a reassuringly familiar look and taste to accompany the new food.

This is a great dish to prepare in advance: store it in the fridge and pop it in the oven when you get home. Double the cooking time (at least) if you're putting this in the oven straight from the fridge.

Vegetables, such as: 5 or 6 large carrots, peeled and cut into bite-size pieces; 5 large potatoes, peeled and thinly sliced; or 1 large or 2 small heads cauliflower, cut into florets
3 tablespoons salted butter, plus 2 tablespoons for topping
3 tablespoons plain flour
480ml milk
½ teaspoon ground black pepper
¼ teaspoon ground nutmeg
1 pinch sea salt, optional
85g dried breadcrumbs
45g grated Parmesan cheese

1. Preheat the oven to 200°C/gas mark 4.
2. In a large saucepan over medium-high heat, bring 1.5 litres of water to a rolling boil. Add the vegetables and cook until crisp-tender, 5 to 7 minutes, depending on the veggie and its cut. (Do not overcook—you don't want mushy veggies.) Drain the vegetables and set aside.
3. Meanwhile, make the white sauce: In a medium saucepan over medium heat, melt 3 tablespoons of butter. Increase the heat to high, add the flour, and cook, whisking vigorously, for 1 minute (make sure the mixture doesn't burn!). Add the milk, reduce the

heat to medium (not too low!), and cook, stirring constantly, for 2 to 3 minutes, just until the sauce begins to thicken. Add the pepper, nutmeg, and salt, if using.

4. Pour the veggies into a baking dish and cover evenly with the sauce. Set aside.

5. In a small bowl, combine the breadcrumbs and Parmesan. Sprinkle the mixture evenly over the top of the casserole. Dot with 2 tablespoons of butter cut into small pieces. Bake in the oven for 8 to 10 minutes, or until the topping is golden brown and crunchy.

Taste-Training Tip: When you first make this dish, use a vegetable your children already like. Once they like the gratin-style, start adding different vegetables. Ask your kids to think of combinations they'd like to try—the possibilities are endless!

Pistou (a.k.a. "Green Ketchup")

Special equipment: food processor or blender
Preparation: 10 minutes
Cooking: 7 minutes
Serving: about 240ml

My kids were the ones who began calling this "green ketchup." It can be used as a dip, a sauce, and a condiment on everything from veggies to pasta!

½ head broccoli, cut into florets
Small handful fresh basil leaves
1 tablespoon extra virgin olive oil
3 teaspoons grated Parmesan cheese

1 tablespoon fresh lemon juice
⅛ teaspoon dried thyme or ¼ teaspoon fresh thyme leaves
60g roasted unsalted sunflower seeds, optional
240ml *Brodo* (page 364) or ready-to-use low-sodium vegetable stock
Sea salt, to taste

1. Bring a medium saucepan of water to a boil over medium heat. Add the broccoli and cook until soft, 7 or 8 minutes. Strain the broccoli, reserving the cooking liquid.

2. In a food processor or blender, combine the cooked broccoli, basil, oil, Parmesan, lemon juice, thyme, sunflower seeds, if using, and 120ml of the broccoli cooking liquid and purée until smooth. Taste and add salt, to taste (I personally don't salt my *pistou*, but some do!) *Pistou* keeps well stored in an airtight container in the fridge for up to a week. I sometimes freeze what I don't use in little ice-cube trays (although this changes the texture slightly); it will keep for up to a month in the freezer.

Notes

Introduction

1. http://mandarine-et-kiwi.blogspot.ca (a French-language blog on "sensory food education" in Canada); Dazeley, P. (2012). Should healthy eating programmes incorporate interaction with foods in different sensory modalities? A review of the evidence. *British Journal of Nutrition* 108(5): 769–77; Dovey, T.M., Aldridge, V.K., Dignan, W., Staples, P.A., Gibson, E.L., and Halford, J.C.G. (2012). Developmental differences in sensory decision making involved in deciding to try a novel fruit. *British Journal of Health Psychology* 17: 258–72; Kannan, S., et al. (2011). "FruitZotic": A sensory approach to introducing preschoolers to fresh exotic fruits at head start locations in western Massachusetts. *Journal of Nutrition Education and Behavior* 43(3): 205–6; Mustonen, S., et al. (2009). Effect of sensory education on school children's food perception: A 2-year follow-up study. *Food Quality and Preference* 20(3): 230–40; Mustonen, S., and Tuorila, H. (2010). Sensory education decreases food neophobia score and encourages trying unfamiliar foods in 8- to 12-year-old children. *Food Quality and Preference* 21(4): 353–60; Reverdy, C., et al. (2008). Effect of sensory education on willingness to taste novel food in children. *Appetite* 51(1): 156–65; Reverdy, C., et al. Effect of sensory education on food preferences in children. *Food Quality and Preference* 21(7): 794–804; Woo, T., and K. Lee. (2011). Development of a sensory education textbook and teaching guidebook for preference improvement toward traditional Korean foods in schoolchildren. *Korean Journal of Nutrition* 44(4): 303–11.

2. The French Ministry of Education guide is available at: http://alimentation.gouv.fr/IMG/pdf/Classesdugout-formationdesenseignants_cle09fcdb.pdf. For more information on the history of "sensory education" in France, see: http://alimentation.gouv.fr/reseau-education-gout.

3. Many of these techniques have also been applied in environmental education (learning about nature, often in outdoor settings). See, for example, Classen, C. (ed.). (2005). *The Book of Touch: Sensory Formations*. Oxford: Berg Publishers; Riener, M. (2009). Sensory cues, visualization and physics learning. *International Journal of Science Education* 31(3): 343–64.

4. Dazeley, P., et al. (2012). Should healthy eating programmes incorporate interaction with foods in different sensory modalities? A review of the evidence. *British Journal of Nutrition* 108(5): 769–77; Dovey, T.M., et al. (2012). Developmental differences in sensory decision making involved in deciding to try a novel fruit. *British Journal of Health Psychology* 17: 258–72; Kannan, S., et al. (2011). "FruitZotic": A sensory approach to introducing preschoolers to fresh exotic fruits at head start locations in Western Massachusetts. *Journal of Nutrition Education and Behavior* 43(3): 205–6; Mustonen, S., et al. (2009). Effect of sensory education on school children's food perception: A 2-year follow-up study. *Food Quality and Preference* 20(3): 230–40; Mustonen, S., and Tuorila, H. (2010). Sensory education decreases food neophobia score and encourages trying unfamiliar foods in 8- to 12-year-old children. *Food Quality and Preference* 21(4): 353–60; Reverdy, C., et. al. (2008). Effect of sensory education on willingness to taste novel food in children. *Appetite* 51(1): 156–65; Reverdy, C., et al. Effect of sensory education on food preferences in children. *Food Quality and Preference* 21(7): 794–804; Woo, T., and K. Lee. (2011). Development of a sensory education textbook and teaching guidebook for preference improvement toward traditional Korean foods in schoolchildren. *Korean Journal of Nutrition* 44(4): 303–11; Rinck, F., et. al. (2011). Ontogeny of odor liking during childhood and its relation to language development. *Chemical Senses* 3(1): 83–91.

5. Rigal, N. (2006). *Winning the Food Fight*. Rochester, VT: Healing Arts Press.

6. See, for example, the joint statement by the Canadian Pediatric

Society and the Canadian Society of Allergy and Clinical Immunology: Chan, E., and Cummings, C. (2013). Dietary exposures and allergy prevention in high-risk infants. *Paediatrics and Child Health* 18(10): 545–49. The American Association of Pediatrics made a similar statement in 2008: Greer, F., et al. (2008). Effects of early nutritional interventions on the development of atopic disease in infants and children: The role of maternal dietary restriction, breastfeeding, timing of introduction of complementary foods, and hydrolyzed formulas. *Pediatrics* 121(1): 183–91. This brings the Canadian and American approaches in line with those in much of Europe.

Secret 1: Kids Can *Learn* to Love Healthy Foods

1. Rosenthal, R., and Jacobson, L. (1969). *Pygmalion in the Classroom: Teacher Expectation and Pupil's Intellectual Development.* New York: Irvington Publishers. See also Rosenthal, R., and Jacobson, L. (1968). Pygmalion in the classroom. *The Urban Review* 3(1): 16–20; and Rosenthal, R. (1994). Interpersonal expectancy effects: A 30-year perspective. *Current Directions in Psychological Science* 3(6): 176–9; Rosenthal, R., and Rubin, D.B. (1978). Interpersonal expectancy effects: The first 345 studies. *Behavioral and Brain Sciences* 1(3): 377–86.

2. Rozin, P., Fallon, A., and Augustoni-Ziskind, M. (1985). The child's conception of food: The development of contamination sensitivity to "disgusting" substances. *Developmental Psychology* 21(6): 1075–9.

3. Birch, L.L. (1980). The relationship between children's food preferences and those of their parents. *Journal of Nutrition Education* 12: 14–18; Birch, L.L. (1999). Development of food preferences. *Annual Review of Nutrition* 19: 41–62; Skinner, J.D., et al. (2002). Children's food preferences: A longitudinal analysis. *Journal of the American Dietetic Association* 102(11): 1638–47.

4. Bartoshuk, L.M. (1991). Sweetness: History, preference, and genetic variability. *Food Technology* 45(11): 108, 110, 112–13; Hayes, J.A., and Keast, R.S.J. (2011). Two decades of supertasting: Where do we stand? *Physiology and Behavior* (104)5: 1072–4; Berridge, K.C. Taste reactivity: Measuring hedonic impact in infants and animals. *Neuroscience and Biobehavioral Reviews* 24: 173–98.

5. Bartoshuk, L.M. (2000). Comparing sensory experiences across individuals: Recent psychophysical advances illuminate genetic variation in taste perception. *Chemical Senses* 25: 447–60; Tepper, B.J. (1999). Does genetic taste sensitivity to PROP influence food preferences and body weight? *Appetite* 32(3): 422.

6. West, C. (2009, July/August). Measuring magnitude. *Observer of the American Association for Psychological Science* 22(6).

7. Duffy, V.B., and Bartoshuk, L.M. (2000). Food acceptance and genetic variation in taste. *Journal of the American Dietetic Association* 100: 647–55; Miller, I.J., and Reedy, F.E. (1990). Variations in human taste bud density and taste intensity perception. *Physiology and Behavior* 47: 1213–19.

8. Bartoshuk, L.M., Duffy, V.B., and Miller, I.J. (1994). PTC/PROP tasting: Anatomy, psychophysics, and sex effects. *Physiology and Behavior* 56: 1165–71.

9. Zeinstra, G., et al. (2009). Facial expressions in school-aged children are a good indicator of "dislikes," but not of "likes." *Food Quality and Preference* 20(8): 620–24.

10. Pliner, P., Pelchat, M., and Grabski, M. (1993). Reduction of neophobia in humans by exposure to novel foods. *Appetite* 20(2): 111–23; Cooke, L. (2007). The importance of exposure for healthy eating in childhood: A review. *Journal of Human Nutrition and Dietetics* 20(4): 294–301.

11. Loewen, R., and Pliner, P. (1999). Effects of prior exposure to palatable and unpalatable novel foods on children's willingness to taste other novel foods. *Appetite* 32(3): 351–66.

12. Birch, L.L., and Marlin, D.F. (1982). I don't like it; I never tried it: Effects of exposure on two-year-old children's food preferences. *Appetite* 3(4): 353–60; Aldridge, V., Dovey, T.M., and Halford, J. (2009). The role of familiarity in dietary development. *Developmental Review* 29(1): 32–44; Cooke, L. (2007). The importance of exposure for healthy eating in childhood: A review. *Journal of Human Nutrition and Dietetics* 20(4): 294–01; Pelchat, M., and Pliner, P. (1995). "Try it. You'll like it": Effects of information on willingness to try novel foods. *Appetite* 24(2): 153–65.

13. Loewen, R., and Pliner, P. (1999). Effects of prior exposure to palatable and unpalatable novel foods on children's willingness to taste other novel foods. *Appetite* 32(3): 351–66.

14. Birch, L.L., et al. (1987). What kind of exposure reduces children's food neophobia? Looking vs. tasting. *Appetite* 9(3): 171–8; Williams, K.E., et al. (2008). Practice does make perfect: A longitudinal look at repeated taste exposure. *Appetite* 51(3): 739–42; Heath, P., Houston-Price, C., and Kennedy, O.B. (2011). Increasing food familiarity without the tears: A role for visual exposure? *Appetite* 57(3): 832–8; Houston-Price, C., Butler, L., and Shiba, P. (2009). Visual exposure impacts on toddlers' willingness to taste fruits and vegetables. *Appetite* 53(3): 450–53.

15. Kessler, D. (2010). *The End of Over-eating: Taking Control of the Insatiable American Appetite.* Emmaus, PA: Rodale Books.

16. Ventura, A., and Mennella, J. (2011). Innate and learned preference for sweet taste during childhood. *Current Opinion in Clinical Nutrition and Metabolic Care* 14(4): 379–84.

17. Harrison, D., et al. (2010). Analgesic effects of sweet-tasting solutions for infants: Current state of equipoise. *Pediatrics* 126(5): 894–902.

18. Baeyens, F., et al. (1990). Flavor-flavor and color-flavor conditioning in humans. *Learning and Motivation* 21(4): 434–55.

19. Eertmans, A., Baeyens, F., and Van den Bergh, O. (2001). Food likes and their relative importance in human eating behavior: Review and preliminary suggestions for health promotion. *Health Education Research: Theory and Practice* 16(4): 443–56.

20. Capaldi, E.D., and Privitera, G.J. (2008). Decreasing dislike for sour and bitter in children and adults. *Appetite* 50(1): 139–45.

21. Havermans, R.C., and Jansen, A. (2007). Increasing children's liking of vegetables through flavour-flavour learning. *Appetite* 48(2): 259–62.

22. Pliner, P., and Stallberg-White, C. (2000). "Pass the ketchup, please": Familiar flavors increase children's willingness to taste novel foods. *Appetite* 34(1): 95–103.

23. Rozin, P. (1976). "The selection of foods by rats, humans, and other animals," in Rosenblatt, J., et al. (eds.), *Advances in the Study of Behavior* (Vol. 6). New York: Academic Press, 21–76.

24. Fallon, A.E., Rozin, P., and Pliner, P. (1984). The child's conception of food: The development of food rejections with special reference to disgust and contamination sensitivity. *Child Development*: 566–75.

25. Miller, G. (2011). Sweet here, salty there: Evidence for a taste map in the mammalian brain. *Science* 333(6047): 1213; Chen, X., et al. (2011). A gustotopic map of taste qualities in the mammalian brain, *Science* 333(6047): 1262–6.

26. Schiffman, S.S. (1997). Taste and smell losses in normal aging and disease. *Journal of the American Medical Association* 278(16): 1357–62.

27. Anzman, S.L., Rollins, B.Y., and Birch, L.L. (2010). Parental influence on children's early eating environments and obesity risk: Implications for prevention. *International Journal of Obesity* 34(7): 1116–24.

Secret 2: Marketing Healthy Food to Your Kids Really Works!

1. Accessed at: http://news.bbc.co.uk/2/hi/uk_news/england/8492477.stm.

2. Accessed at: http://www.primaryindustrieseducation.com.au/resources/reports/foodfibrefuture.pdf.

3. Howden, N. (2012, March 5). Cultural cringe: Schoolchildren can't see the yoghurt for the trees. *Sydney Morning Herald*. See also Hillman, K., and Buckley, S. (2011). Food, fibre, and the future: Report on surveys of students' and teachers' knowledge and understanding of Primary Industries. *Report to the Australian Council for Educational Research*. Sydney: ACER. Accessed at: http://www.primaryindustrieseducation.com.au/resources/reports/foodfibrefuture.pdf.

4. Schor, J.B., and Ford, M. (2007). From tastes great to cool: Children's food marketing and the rise of the symbolic. *The Journal of Law, Medicine and Ethics* 35(1): 10–21; Desrochers, D.M., and Holt, D.J. (2007). Children's exposure to television advertising: Implications for childhood obesity. *Journal of Public Policy and Marketing* 26(2): 20; Dorfman, L.E., and Wootan, M.G. (2012). The nation needs to do more to address food marketing to children. *American Journal of Preventive Medicine* 42(3): 334; Cairns, G., et al. (2013). Systematic reviews of the evidence on the nature, extent and effects of food marketing to children: A retrospective summary. *Appetite* 62: 209–15; Nestle, M. (2002). *Food Politics: How the Food Industry Influences Nutrition, and Health*. Berkeley: University of California Press.

5. Mello, M.M., Studdert, D.M., and Brennan, T.A. (2006). Obesity: The new frontier of public health law. *New England Journal of Medicine* 354(24): 2601–10; Batada, A., et al. (2008). Nine out of 10 food advertisements shown during Saturday morning children's television programming are for foods high in fat, sodium, or added sugars, or low in nutrients. *Journal of the American Dietetic Association* 108(4): 673–8.

6. Harris, J.L., Bargh, J.A., and Brownell. K.D. (2009). Priming effects of television food advertising on eating behavior. *Health Psychology* 28(4): 404–13; Harris, J.L., et al. (2009). A crisis in the marketplace: How food marketing contributes to childhood obesity and what can be done. *Annual Review of Public Health* 30(1): 211–25.

7. Alvy, L., and Calvert, S. (2008). Food marketing on popular children's websites: A content analysis. *Journal of the American Dietetic Association* 108(4): 710–13.

8. Troianovski, A. (2012, March). Child's play: Food makers hook kids on mobile games. *Wall Street Journal*. Accessed at: http://online.wsj.com/news/articles/SB1000087239639044481270457760 5263654758948.

9. BBC News Online. (2011, December 17). Food firms market to children online. Accessed at: http://www.bbc.co.uk/news/health-16217306.

10. Richtel, M. (2011, April 20). In online games: A path to young consumers. *The New York Times*. Accessed at: http://www.nytimes.com/2011/04/21/business/21marketing.html?pagewanted=all&_r=0.

11. von Normann, K. (2009). The impact of lifestyles and food knowledge on the food patterns of German children. *International Journal of Consumer Studies* 33(4): 382–91; Harris, J.L., Brownell, K.D., and Bargh, J.A. (2009). The food marketing defense model: Integrating psychological research to protect youth and inform public policy. *Social Issues and Policy Review* 3(1): 211–71; Chaplin, L.N., and John, D.R. (2005). The development of self-brand connections in children and adolescents. *Journal of Consumer Research* 32: 119–29.

12. Forman, N., et al. (2009). Food branding influences ad libitum intake differently in children depending on weight status: Results of a pilot study. *Appetite* 53(1): 76–83; Nestle, M. (2006). Food marketing and childhood obesity: A matter of policy. *New England Journal of Medicine* 354(24): 2527–9; Nestle, M. (2002).

Food Politics: How the Food Industry Influences Nutrition and Health. Berkeley: University of California Press.

13. McGinnis, J.M., Gootman, J.A., Kraak, V.I. (eds.) (2006). *Food Marketing to Children and Youth: Threat or Opportunity?* Washington, D.C.: National Academies Press.

14. Deliza, R., and MacFie, H.J.H. (1996). The generation of sensory expectation by external cues and its effect on sensory perception and hedonic ratings: A review. *Journal of Sensory Studies* 11: 103–28; Fazio, R.H. (2001). On the automatic activation of associated evaluations: An overview. *Cognition and Emotion* 15: 115–41; Chartrand, T.L., et al. (2008). Nonconscious goals and consumer choice. *Journal of Consumer Research* 35: 189–201.

15. Bargh, J.A., and Ferguson, M.J. (2000). Beyond behaviorism: The automaticity of higher mental processes. *Psychological Bulletin,* 126: 925–45; Strack, F., and Deutsch, R. (2004). Reflective and impulsive determinants of social behavior. *Personality and Social Psychology Review* 8: 220–47; Wilson, T.D., and Bar-Anan, Y. (2008). The unseen mind. *Science* 321: 1046–7; Dijksterhuis, A., Chartrand, T.L., and Aarts, H. (2007). Automatic behavior. In J. A. Bargh (ed.), *Social Psychology and the Unconscious: The Automaticity of Higher Mental Processes.* Philadelphia: Psychology Press. Similar findings hold true for young children's perceptions of alcohol consumption, see: Austin, E.W., and Knaus, C. (2000). Predicting the potential for risky behavior among those "too young" to drink as the result of appealing advertising. *Journal of Health Communication* 5: 13–27. This is also why traditional "exercise more" or "eat healthy" messages from public health providers have been shown to be relatively ineffective in changing long-term behaviors. See, for example, Wardle, J., and Huon, G. (2000). An experimental investigation of the influence of health information on children's taste preferences. *Health Education Research* 15: 39–44.

16. Schor, J.B., and Ford, M. (2007). From tastes great to cool: Children's food marketing and the rise of the symbolic. *Journal of Law, Medicine and Ethics* 35: 10–21.

17. Nestle, M. (2002). *Food Politics: How the Food Industry Influences Nutrition, and Health.* Berkeley: University of California Press.

18. Christakis, D.A. (2008). The effects of infant media usage: What do we know and what should we learn? *Acta Paediatrica* 98(1): 8–16; Lillard, A.S., and Peterson, J. (2011). The immediate impact of different types of television on young children's executive function. *Pediatrics* 128(4): 644–9; Zimmerman, F.J., Christakis, D.A., and Meltzoff, A.N. (2007). Associations between media viewing and language development in children under age 2 years. *Journal of Pediatrics* 151(4): 364–68; Page, A., et al. (2010). Children's screen viewing is related to psychological difficulties irrespective of physical activity. *Pediatrics.* doi: 10.1542/peds. 2010–1154; Strasburger, V.C., et al. (2011). Policy statement: Children, adolescents, obesity, and the media. *Pediatrics* 128: 201–8; Boyland, E.J., et al. (2011). Food commercials increase preference for energy-dense foods, particularly in children who watch more television. *Pediatrics* 128: e93–e100.

19. Halford, J.C.G., et al. (2004). Effect of television advertisements for foods on food consumption in children. *Appetite* 42: 221–5; Halford, J.C.G., et al. (2007). Beyond-brand effect of television (TV) food advertisement/commercials on caloric intake and food choice of 5- to 7-year-old children. *Appetite* 49: 263–7; Harris, J.L., Bargh, J.A., and Brownell, K. (2009). The direct effects of television food advertising on eating behavior. *Health Psychology* 28: 404–13.

20. Wansink, B., et al. (2012). Attractive names sustain increased vegetable intake in schools. *Preventive Medicine* 55(4): 330–32; Wansink, B., et al. (2011).What is in a name? Giving descriptive names to vegetables increases lunchroom sales. *Journal of Nutrition Education and Behavior* 43(4): S1.

21. Wansink, B., et al. (2012). Can branding improve school lunches? *Preventive Medicine* 166(10): 967–8.

22. Wansink, B., Shimizu, M., Camps, G. (2011). What would Batman eat?: Priming children to make healthier fast food choices. *Pediatric Obesity* 7: 121–3.

23. Morizet, D., et al. (2012). Effect of labeling on new vegetable dish acceptance in preadolescent children. *Appetite* 59(2): 399–402.

24. Harper, L., and Sanders, K. (1975). The effect of adults' eating on young childrens' acceptance of unfamiliar foods. *Journal of Experimental Child Psychology* 20: 200–14; Hendy, H., and Raudenbush, B. (2000). Effectiveness of teacher modeling to

encourage food acceptance in preschool children. *Appetite* 34(1): 61–76; Jansen, A., and Tenney, N. (2001). Seeing mum drinking a "light" product: Is social learning a stronger determinant of taste preference acquisition than caloric conditioning? *European Journal of Clinical Nutrition* 55(6): 418–22.

25. L.L. Birch. (1980). Effects of peer models' food choices and eating behaviours on preschoolers' food preferences. *Child Development* 51: 489–96.

26. French, S.A., et al. (1999). Cognitive and demographic correlates of low-fat vending snack choices among adolescents and adults. *Journal of the American Dietetic Association* 99(4): 471–5; Zandstra, E.H., De Graaf, C., and Van Staveren, W. (2001). Influence of health and taste attitudes on consumption of low- and high-fat foods. *Food Quality and Preference* 12: 75–82; Glanz, K., et al. (1998). Why Americans eat what they do: Taste, nutrition, cost, convenience and weight control concerns as influences on food consumption. *Journal of the American Dietetic Association* 98: 1118–26; Neumark-Sztainer, D., et al. (2003). Correlates of fruit and vegetable intake among adolescents: Findings from Project EAT. *Preventive Medicine* 37: 198–208.

27. Kitts, D. (1994). Bioactive substances in food: Identification and potential uses. *Canadian Journal of Physiology and Pharmacology* 72: 423–34.

28. Cooke, L.J. et al. (2011). Eating for pleasure or profit. *Psychological Science* 22(2): 190–96.

29. Sekar, R., Rajagopal, P., and Gilbride, T.J. (2010). Marketing healthful eating to children: The effectiveness of incentives, pledges, and competitions. *Journal of Marketing* 74(3): 93–106.

30. These were tried in a *Consumer Reports* blind taste test of 19 different product pairs, which found little significant taste differences in these instances. In each of these cases, the *Consumer Reports* testers found little or no difference in the taste quality of the name brand versus store-bought foods. *Consumer Reports.* (2012, October). Store-brand vs. name-brand taste-off: Our tests pit private-label products against big-name rivals. Accessed at: http://consumerreports.org/cro/magazine/2012/10/store-brand-vs-name-brand-taste-off/index.htm.

31. Robinson, T.N., et al. (2007). Effects of fast food branding on young children's taste preferences. *Archives of Pediatric and*

Adolescent Medicine 161: 792–7.

32. Moore, E.S., and Lutz, R.L. (2000). Children, advertising, and product experiences: A multimethod inquiry. *Journal of Consumer Research* 27: 31–48.

33. Raju, S., et al. (2010). Marketing healthful eating to children: The effectiveness of incentives, pledges, and competitions. *Journal of Marketing* 74(3): 93–106.

34. Cooke, L.J. et al. (2011). Eating for pleasure or profit. *Psychological Science* 22(2): 190–96.

Secret 3: Schedule One Snack a Day

1. Waller, C.E., Du, S., and Popkin, B.M. (2012). Patterns of over-weight, inactivity, and snacking in Chinese children. *Obesity Research* 11(8): 957–61.

2. Piernas, C., and Popkin, B.M. (2010). Trends in snacking among US children. *Health Affairs*, 29(3): 398–404.

3. See http://www.letsmove.gov.

4. Piernas, C., and Popkin, B.M. (2010). Snacking increased among US adults between 1977 and 2006. *Journal of Nutrition* 140(2): 325–32.

5. Kerr, M.A., et al. (2009). Snacking patterns among adolescents: A comparison of type, frequency and portion size between Britain in 1997 and Northern Ireland in 2005. *British Journal of Nutrition* 101(1): 122.

6. Jahns, L., Siega-Riz, A.M., and Popkin, B.M. (2001). The increasing prevalence of snacking among US children from 1977 to 1996. *The Journal of Pediatrics* 138(4): 493–8; Zizza, C., Siega-Riz, A.M., and Popkin, B.M. (2001). Significant increase in young adults' snacking between 1977–1978 and 1994–1996 represents a cause for concern! *Preventive Medicine* 32(4): 303–10.

7. Kessler, D. (2009). *The End of Over-eating: Taking Control of the Insatiable American Appetite.* Emmaus, PA: Rodale Press.

8. Fisher, J.O., and Birch, L.L. (2002). Eating in the absence of hunger and overweight in girls from 5 to 7 years of age. *American Journal of Clinical Nutrition* 76(1): 226–31.

9. Kagamimori, S., et al. (2008). The relationship between lifestyle, social characteristics, and obesity in 3-year-old Japanese children. *Child: Care, Health and Development* 25(3): 235–48.

10. Abramson, E. (2011). *It's Not Just Baby Fat.* n.p.: Bodega Books.

11. Birch, L.L., and Deysher, M. (1985). Conditioned and unconditioned caloric compensation: Evidence for self-regulation of food intake by young children. *Learning and Motivation* 16: 341–55; Deysher, M. (1986). Caloric compensation and sensory specific satiety: Evidence for self-regulation of food intake by young children. *Appetite* 7(4): 323–31.

12. Young, L.R., and Nestle, M. (2003). Expanding portion sizes in the U.S. marketplace: Implications for nutrition counseling. *Journal of the American Dietetic Association* 103(2): 231–4.

13. Mischel, W., et al. (1972). Cognitive and attentional mechanisms in delay of gratification. *Journal of Personality and Social Psychology* 21(2): 204–18. See also: Eigste, I., et al. (2006). Predicting cognitive control from preschool to late adolescence and young adulthood. *Psychological Science* 17(6): 478–84; Casey, B. J., et al. (2011, August 29). Behavioral and neural correlates of delay of gratification 40 years later. *Proceedings of the National Academy of Sciences* u108(36): 14998–15003.

14. Honkanen, P., et al. (2012). Reflective and impulsive influences on unhealthy snacking: The moderating effects of food-related self-control. *Appetite* 58(2): 616–22.

15. Flood-Obbagy, J.E., and Rolls, B.J. (2009). The effect of fruit in different forms on energy intake and satiety at a meal. *Appetite* 52(2): 416–22.

16. Cornwell, T.B., and McAlister, A.R. (2012). Contingent choice: Exploring the relationship between sweetened beverages and vegetable consumption. *Appetite* 62: 203–8. doi: http://dx.doi.org/10.1016/j.appet.2012.05.001.

17. Cheng, J. (2012). Food for thought. *Journal of the American Medical Association* 308(11): 1101–2.

18. Adapted from the French Ministry of Education guide, available at: http://alimentation.gouv.fr/IMG/pdf/Classesdugout-formationdesenseignants_cle09fcdb.pdf.

19. Gori, M., et al. (2008). Young children do not integrate visual and haptic form information. *Current Biology* 18(9): 694–8.

20. Lukasewycz, L.D., and Mennella, J.A. (2012). Lingual tactile acuity and food texture preferences among children and their mothers. *Food Quality and Preference* 26(1): 58–66.

Secret 4: Routines and Rituals Make Healthy Eating Automatic (and Fun!)

1. Spill, M., et al. (2010). Eating vegetables first: The use of portion size to increase vegetable consumption in preschool children. *American Journal of Clinical Nutrition* 91(5): 1237–43; Wardle, J., et al. (2012). Parental feeding style and the inter-generational transmission of obesity risk. *Obesity Research* 10(6): 453–62.

2. Birch, L.L. (1980). The relationship between children's food preferences and those of their parents. *Journal of Nutrition Education* 12: 14–18.

3. Morizet, D., et. al. (2011). Perceptual and lexical knowledge of vegetables in preadolescent children. *Appetite* 56(1): 142–7.

4. Shutts, K., et al. (2009). Social information guides infants' selection of foods. *Journal of Cognition and Development* 10(1–2): 1–17; Stevenson, R., et al. (2010). Children's response to adult disgust elicitors: Development and acquisition. *Developmental Psychology* 46(1): 165–77.

5. Greenhalgh, J., et al. (2009). Positive and negative peer modeling effects on young children's consumption of novel blue foods. *Appetite* 52(3): 646–53.

6. Horne, P.J., et al. (2008). Increasing parental provision and children's consumption of lunchbox fruit and vegetables in Ireland: The Food Dudes intervention. *European Journal of Clinical Nutrition* 63(5): 613–18; Horne, P.J., et al. (1995). An effective procedure for changing food preferences in 5- to 7-year-old children. *Proceedings of the Nutrition Society* 54(2): 441–52.

7. Rozin, P., and Nemeroff, C.J. (1990). The laws of sympathetic magic: A psychological analysis of similarity and contagion. In Stigler, J., Herdt, G., and Shweder, R.A. (eds.), *Cultural Psychology: Essays on Comparative Human Development.* Cambridge, UK: Cambridge University Press, 205–32.

8. Ochs, E., and Shohet, M. (2006). The cultural structuring of mealtime socialization. *New Directions for Child and Adolescent Development* 111: 35–49.

Secret 5: Kids Don't Need Kids' Food

1. Moriyama, N. (2005). *Japanese Women Don't Get Old or Fat.* Guilford, UK: Delta.

2. Rose, D. (2012, March 15). Blog post: The truth about kid-friendly

foods. Accessed at: www.psychologytoday.com/blog/the-art-science-teaching-kids-right/201203/the-truth-about-child-friendly-foods; Kessler, D. (2009). *The End of Over-Eating: Taking Control of the Insatiable American Appetite*. Emmaus, PA: Rodale Press.

3. Burger, K.S., and Stice, E. (2012). Frequent ice cream consumption is associated with reduced striatal response to receipt of an ice cream–based milkshake. *American Journal of Clinical Nutrition* 95(4): 810–17.

4. Kessler, D. (2009). *The End of Over-Eating: Taking Control of the Insatiable American Appetite*. Emmaus, PA: Rodale Press.

5. Johnson, P., and Kenny, P. (2010). Dopamine D2 receptors in addiction-like reward dysfunction and compulsive eating in obese rats. *Nature Neuroscience* 13: 635–41; Epstein, D., and Shaham, Y. (2010). Cheesecake-eating rats and the question of food addiction. *Nature Neuroscience* 13: 529–31.

6. Rose, D. (2012, March 15). Blog post: The truth about kid-friendly foods. Accessed at: www.psychologytoday.com/blog/the-art-science-teaching-kids-right/201203/the-truth-about-child-friendly-foods.

7. Kessler, D. (2009). *The End of Over-eating: Taking Control of the Insatiable American Appetite*. Emmaus, PA: Rodale Press.

8. Accessed at: http://www.cancer.umn.edu/research/programs/peiowa.html.

9. Fisher, J.O., and Birch, L.L. (1999). Restricting access to palatable foods affects children's behavioral response, food selection, and intake. *American Journal of Clinical Nutrition* 69(6): 1264–72.

10. Addessi, E., et al. (2005). Specific social influences on the acceptance of novel foods in 2- to 5-year-old children. *Appetite* 45(3): 264–71; Haire-Joshu, D., et al. (2008). High 5 for kids: The impact of a home visiting program on fruit and vegetable intake of parents and their preschool children. *Preventative Medicine* 47(1): 77–8; Hughes, S.O., et al. (2007). The impact of childcare providers' feeding on children's food consumption. *Journal of Developmental and Behavioral Pediatrics* 28(2): 100–107; Wardle, J., Carnell, S., and Cooke, L. (2005). Parental control over feeding and children's fruit and vegetable intake: How are they related? *Journal of the American Dietetic Association* 105(2): 227–32.

11. Bittman, M. (2012, June). Which diet works? *New York Times*. Accessed at: http://opinionator.blogs.nytimes.com/2012/06/26/which-diet-works/?hp.

12. Cooper, E. (1986). Chinese table manners: You are how you eat. *Human Organization* 45(2): 179–84.

13. Birch, L.L., et al. 1987. What kind of exposure reduces children's food neophobia? Looking vs. tasting. *Appetite* 9(3): 171–8.

14. Busick, D.B., et al. (2008, November). Parent food purchases as a measure of exposure and preschool-aged children's willingness to identify and taste fruit and vegetables. *Appetite* 51(3): 468–73; Wardle, J., et al. (2003a). Increasing children's acceptance of vegetables: A randomized trial of parent-led exposure. *Appetite* 40(2): 155–62; Wardle, J., et al. (2003b). Modifying children's food preferences: The effects of exposure and reward on acceptance of an unfamiliar vegetable. *European Journal of Clinical Nutrition* 57(2): 341–8.

15. Wardle, J., et al. (2003a). Increasing children's acceptance of vegetables: A randomized trial of parent-led exposure. *Appetite* 40(2): 155–62; Wardle, J., et al. (2003b). Modifying children's food preferences: The effects of exposure and reward on acceptance of an unfamiliar vegetable. *European Journal of Clinical Nutrition* 57(2): 341–8.

16. Howard, A.J., et al. (2012). Toddlers' food preferences: The impact of novel food exposure, maternal preferences, and food neophobia. *Appetite* 59(3): 818–25.

17. Ministère de l'Éducation Nationale. (2012). *Programme de formation des enseignants sur les classes du goût.* Paris: French National Ministry of Education.

18. McCrickerd, K., et al. (2012). Subtle changes in the flavour and texture of a drink enhance expectations of satiety. *Appetite* 59(2): 632.

19. Johnson, J., and Clydesdale, F.M. (1982). Perceived sweetness and redness in colored sucrose solutions. *Journal of Food Science* 47: 747–52.

20. The Centre for Science in the Public Interest has an excellent online resource that explains the health risks of different food additives, see: http://www.cspinet.org/reports/chemcuisine.htm.

21. Sinn, N. (2008). Nutritional and dietary influences on attention deficit hyperactivity disorder. *Nutrition Reviews* 66(10): 558–68; McCann, D., et al. Food additives and hyperactive behavior in 3-year-old and 8-/9-year-old children in the community: A randomised, double-blinded, placebo-controlled trial. *Lancet* 370(9598): 1560–67.

22. Weiss, B. (2010). Synthetic food colors and neurobehavioral hazards: The view from environmental health research. *Environmental Health Perspectives* 120(1): 1.

Secret 6: Participation Works Better than Pressure

1. Carper, J.L., Fisher, J.O., and Birch, L.L. (2000). Young girl's emerging dietary restraint and disinhibition are related to parental control in child feeding. *Appetite* 35(2): 121–9.
2. Jansen, E., Mulkens, S., and Jansen, A. (2007). Do not eat the red food!: Prohibition of snacks leads to their relatively higher consumption in children. *Appetite* 49(3): 572–7.
3. Nanney, M.S., et al. (2007). Frequency of eating homegrown produce is associated with higher intake among parents and their preschool-aged children in rural Missouri. *Journal of the American Dietetic Association* 107(4): 577–84; Heim, S., et al. (2011). Can a community-based intervention improve the home food environment? Parental perspectives of the influence of the delicious and nutritious garden. *Journal of Nutrition Education and Behavior* 43(2): 130–34; Somerset, S., and Markwell, K. (2009). Impact of a schoolbased food garden on attitudes and identification skills regarding vegetables and fruit: A 12-month intervention trial. *Public Health Nutrition* 12: 214–21; Parmer, S.M., et al. (2009). School gardens: An experiential learning approach for a nutrition education program to increase fruit and vegetable knowledge, preference, and consumption among second-grade students. *Journal of Nutrition Education and Behavior* 41: 212–17.

Secret 7: Mindful Eating Is Mealtime Magic

1. Wansink, B., Painter, J.E., and North, J. (2005). Bottomless bowls: Why visual cues of portion size may influence intake. *Obesity Research* 13(1): 93–100.
2. Accessed at: http://foodpsychology.cornell.edu/outreach/bottomless-bowls.html.
3. Wansink, B. (2004). Environmental factors that unknowingly increase a consumer's food intake and consumption volume. *Annual Review of Nutrition* 24: 455–79; Wansink, B., Van Ittersum, K., and Painter, J.E. (2006). Ice cream illusions: Bowls, spoons, and self-served portion sizes. *American Journal of Preventive Medicine* 31(3): 240–43; Wansink, B., and Kim, J. (2005). Bad popcorn in

big buckets: Portion size can influence intake as much as taste. *Journal of Nutrition Education and Behavior* 37(5): 242–5; Wansink, B., and Cheney, M.M. (2005). Super bowls: Serving bowl size and food consumption. *JAMA* 293(14): 1727–8.

4. Marteau, T.M., Hollands, G.H., and Fletcher, P.C. (2012). Changing human behavior to prevent disease: The importance of targeting automatic processes. *Science* 337(6101): 1492–5.

5. Hanks, A., Just, D., and Wansink, B. (2012). Trigger foods: The influence of "irrelevant" alternatives in school lunchrooms. *Agricultural and Resource Economics Review* 41(1): 114–23.

6. Halford, J.C.G. (2012). Developmental differences in sensory decision making involved in deciding to try a novel fruit. *British Journal of Health Psychology* 17: 258–72.

7. Hill, J.O., and Peters, J.C. (1998). Environmental contributions to the obesity epidemic. *Science* 280: 1371–4.

8. Accessed at: http://mindlesseating.org/faq.php.

9. Accessed at: http://www.suntimes.com/lifestyles/food/16808808-423/cooking-for-kids-sweet.html.

10. Howard, A.J., et al. (2012). Toddlers' food preferences: The impact of novel food exposure, maternal preferences and food neophobia. *Appetite* 59(3): 818–25.

11. Fischler, C. *L'homnivore*. Paris: Odile Jacob.

12. Beltran, A., et al. (2011). Identifying and clarifying values and reason statements that promote effective food parenting practices, using intensive interviews. *Journal of Nutrition Education and Behavior* 43(6): 531–5

13. Bone, J. (2005). Breaking bread: Spirituality, food and early childhood education. *International Journal of Children's Spirituality* 10(3): 307–17; Nath, J. (2010). God is a vegetarian: The food, health and bio-spirituality of Hare Krishna, Buddhist, and Seventh-Day Adventist devotees. *Health Sociology Review* 19(3): 356–68.

14. Kleef, E.V., Shimizu, M., and Wansink, B. (2012). Just a bite: Considerably smaller snack portions satisfy delayed hunger and craving. *Food Quality and Preference* 27(1): 96–100.

15. Birch, L.L. (1980). The relationship between children's food preferences and those of their parents. *Journal of Nutrition Education* 12: 14–18; Wansink, B., Payne, C.R., and Chandon, P. (2007). Internal and external cues of meal cessation: The French paradox redux? *Obesity* 15: 2920–24.

16. CSPI. (2012). *Liquid candy: How soft drinks are harming America's health*. Washington: Centre for Science in the Public Interest.
17. Batsell, W.R., Brown, A.S., Ansfield, A.E., and Paschall, G.Y. (2002). You will eat all of that!: A retrospective analysis of forced consumption episodes. *Appetite* 38(3): 211–19; Brown, K.A., et al. (2008). The role of parental control practices in explaining children's diet and BMI. *Appetite* 50(2–3): 252–9; Galloway, A. (2006). "Finish your soup": Counterproductive effects of pressuring children to eat on intake and affect. *Appetite* 46(3): 318–23.

Babies: Feeding Maximum Variety with Minimum Fuss

1. Birch, L. (1998). Development of food acceptance patterns in the first years of life. *Proceedings of the Nutrition Society* 57(4): 617–24; Birch, L. (1999). Development of food preferences. *Annual Review of Nutrition* 19: 41–62; Mennella, J., et al. (2008). Variety is the spice of life: Strategies for promoting fruit and vegetable acceptance during infancy. *Physiology and Behavior* 94(1): 29–38; Maier, A. (2008). *L'expérience précoce de la variété sensorielle et ses conséquences sur l'alimentation future. Enfance* 60(3): 231–40; Schwartz, C., Issanchou, S., and Nicklaus, S. (2009). Developmental changes in the acceptance of the five basic tastes in the first year of life. *British Journal of Nutrition* 102(9): 1375–85; Schwartz, C., et al. (2010). *A quelles saveurs les nourrissons sont-ils exposés dans la première année de vie? Archives de Pédiatrie* 17(7): 1026–34; Schwartz, C., et al. (2011). The role of taste on food acceptance at weaning. *Physiology and Behaviour* 104: 646–52.
2. Mennella, J.A., et al. (2005). Infant feeding practices and early flavor experiences in Mexican infants: An intra-cultural study. *Journal of the American Dietetic Association* 105(6): 908–15; Birch, L.L., et al. (1998). Infants' consumption of a new food enhances acceptance of similar foods. *Appetite* 30(3): 283–95; Forestell, C.A., and Mennella, J.A. (2007). Early determinants of fruit and vegetable acceptance. *Pediatrics* 120(6): 1247–54.
3. Berkowitz, R.I., et al. (2005). Growth of children at high risk of obesity during the first 6 years of life: Implications for prevention. *American Journal of Clinical Nutrition* 81(1): 140–46; Stettler, N., et al. (2003). Rapid weight gain during infancy and obesity in

young adulthood in a cohort of African Americans. *American Journal of Clinical Nutrition* 77(6): 1374–8; Stunkard, A.J., et al. (2004). Predictors of body size in the first 2 years of life: A high-risk study of human obesity. *International Journal of Obesity and Related Metabolic Disorders* 28(4): 503–13; Whitaker, R.C., et al. (1998). Early adiposity rebound and the risk of adult obesity. *Pediatrics* 101(3): E5.

4. Butte, N., et al. (2004). The start healthy feeding guidelines for infants and toddlers. *Journal of the American Dietetic Association* 104(3): 442 R.I. 54.

5. Dixon, K. (2008, October). Momma, I'll have some of whatever you're having. *New York Times*. Accessed at: http://www.nytimes.com/2008/10/01/dining/01baby.html?pagewanted=printand_r=0.

6. See, for example, Mennella, J.A., and Beauchamp, G.K. (2005). Understanding the origin of flavor preferences. *Chemical Senses* 30 (Supplement): 242–3; Schaal, B., Marlier, L., and Soussignan, R. (2000). Human foetuses learn odours from their pregnant mother's diet. *Chemical Senses* 25: 729–37; Domínguez, P. (2011). The study of postnatal and later development of the taste and olfactory systems using the human brain mapping approach: An update. *Brain Research Bulletin* 84(2): 118–24.

7. See, for example, Mennella, J. (2009). Flavor programming during breastfeeding. *Advances in Experimental Medicine and Biology* 639: 113–20; Gerrish, C.J., and Mennella, J.A. (2001). Flavor variety enhances food acceptance in formula-fed infants. *American Journal of Clinical Nutrition* 73(6): 1080–85; Schwartz, C., et al. (2010). À quelles saveurs les nourrissons sont-ils exposés dans la première année de vie? *Archives de Pédiatrie* 17(7): 1026–34; Nicklaus, S., et al. (2005). A prospective study of food variety-seeking in childhood: Adolescence and early adult life. *Appetite* 44(3): 288–97.

8. Gerrish, C.J., and Mennella, J.A. (2001). Flavor variety enhances food acceptance in formula-fed infants. *The American Journal of Clinical Nutrition* 73(6): 1080–85; Mennella, J.A., Kennedy, J.M., and Beauchamp, G.K. (2006). Vegetable acceptance by infants: Effects of formula flavors. *Early Human Development* 82(7): 463–8.

9. Birch, L.L. (1999). Development of food preferences. *Annual Review of Nutrition* 19: 41–62; Rozin, P., and Millman, L. (1987).

Family environment, not heredity, accounts for family resemblances in food preferences and attitudes: A twin study. *Appetite* 8: 125–34.

10. Maier, A., et al. (2007). Food-related sensory experience from birth through weaning: Contrasted patterns in two nearby European regions. *Appetite* 49: 429–40.

11. Dixon, K. (2008, October). Momma, I'll have some of whatever you're having. *New York Times*. Accessed at: http://www.nytimes.com/2008/10/01/dining/01baby.html?pagewanted=printand_r=0.

12. Accessed at: http://patiented.aap.org/content2.aspx?aid=5713.

13. Ludwig, D. (2007). *Ending the Food Fight: Guide Your Child to a Healthy Weight in a Fast Food/Fake Food World*. Chicago: Houghton Mifflin; Szabo, L. (2010, November). Get the white out of baby's first foods, pediatrician says. *USA Today*. Accessed at: http://usatoday30.usatoday.com/yourlife/parenting-family/babies/2010-12-01-babyfood01_st_N.htm.

14. Sun, Q., et al. (2010, June). White rice, brown rice, and risk of type 2 diabetes in US men and women. *Archives of Internal Medicine* 170(11): 961–9.

15. Butte, N., et al. (2010). Nutrient intakes of US infants, toddlers, and preschoolers meet or exceed dietary reference intakes. *Journal of the American Dietetic Association* (110)12: S27–37 (Supplement).

16. Fox, M.K., et al. (2004, January). Feeding infants and toddlers study: What foods are infants and toddlers eating? *Journal of the American Dietetic Association* 104(1S): 22–30.

17. Bayol, S.A., et al. (2008). Offspring from mothers fed a junk food diet in pregnancy and lactation exhibit exacerbated adiposity which is more pronounced in females. *Journal of Physiology*. doi: 10.1113/jphysiol.2008.153817.

18. Shutts, K., et. al. (2009). Core knowledge and its limits: The domain of food. *Cognition* 112(1): 120–40.

19. Hendy, H.M. (2002). Effectiveness of trained peer models to encourage food acceptance in preschool children. *Appetite* 39(3): 217–25.

20. Rozin, P., Fallon, A., and Augustoni-Ziskind, M. (1985). The child's conception of food: The development of contamination sensitivity to "disgusting" substances. *Developmental Psychology* 21(6): 1075; Fallon, A.E., Rozin, P., and Pliner, P. (1984). The

child's conception of food: The development of food rejections with special reference to disgust and contamination sensitivity. *Child Development*: 566–75.

21. Birch, L.L., and Fisher, J.O. (1998). Development of eating behaviors among children and adolescents. *Pediatrics* 101(Supplement 2): 539–49.

22. Musher-Eizenman, D.R., et al. (2009). Child and parent characteristics related to parental feeding practices: A cross-cultural examination in the US and France. *Appetite* 52(1): 89–95; de Lauzon-Guillain, B., et al. (2009). Parental feeding practices in the United States and in France: Relationships with child's characteristics and parent's eating behavior. *Journal of the American Dietetic Association* 109(6): 1064–6.

23. Hittner, J., and Faith, M. (2011). Typology of emergent eating patterns in early childhood. *Eating Behaviors* 12(4): 242–8; Carnell, S., and Wardle, J. (2008). Appetite and adiposity in children: Evidence for a behavioral susceptibility theory of obesity. *American Journal of Clinical Nutrition* 88(1): 22–9; Wardle, J., et al. (2008). Evidence for a strong genetic influence on childhood adiposity despite the force of the obesogenic environment. *American Journal of Clinical Nutrition* 87(2): 398–404; Ashcroft, J., et al. (2007). Continuity and stability of eating behaviour traits in children. *European Journal of Clinical Nutrition* 62(8): 985–90.

24. Birch, L.L. (1979). Preschool children's preferences and consumption patterns. *Journal of Nutrition Education* 11: 189–92; Birch, L.L., et al. (1987). What kind of exposure reduces children's food neophobia?: Looking vs. tasting. *Appetite* 9(3): 171–8; Birch, L.L. (1990). Development of food acceptance patterns. *Developmental Psychology* 26(4): 515; Birch, L.L. (1999). Development of food preferences. *Annual Review of Nutrition* 19: 41–62; Birch, L.L., and Marlin, D.W. (1982). I don't like it; I never tried it: Effects of exposure on two-year-old children's food preferences. *Appetite* 3(4): 353–60.

25. Birch, L.L., and Fisher, J.O. (1998). Development of eating behaviors among children and adolescents. *Pediatrics* 101(Supplement 2): 539–49.

26. Hittner, J., and Faith, M. (2011). Typology of emergent eating patterns in early childhood. *Eating Behaviors* 12(4): 242–8;

Bartoshuk, L.M., Duffy, V.B., and Miller, I. J. (1994). PTC/PROP tasting: Anatomy, psychophysics, and sex effects. *Physiology and Behavior* 56(6): 1165–71; Bartoshuk, L.M. (2000). Comparing sensory experiences across individuals: Recent psychophysical advances illuminate genetic variation in taste perception. *Chemical Senses* 25(4): 447–60; Tepper, B.J. (1999). Does genetic taste sensitivity to PROP influence food preferences and body weight? *Appetite* 32: 422.

27. Dovey, T.M., et al. (2008). Food neophobia and "picky/fussy" eating in children: A review. *Appetite* 50(2): 181–93; Galloway, A.T., et al. (2006). "Finish your soup": Counterproductive effects of pressuring children to eat on intake and affect. *Appetite* 46(3): 318–23; Pliner, P., and Loewen, E. (1997). Temperament and food neophobia in children and their mothers. *Appetite* 28(3): 239–54; Pliner, P. (1994). Development of measures of food neophobia in children. *Appetite* 23(2): 147–63.

Toddlers: Preventing and Solving Common Eating Challenges

1. Baxter, I.A., Jack, F.R., and Schröder, M. (1998). The use of repertory grid method to elicit perceptual data from primary school children. *Food Quality and Preference* 9(1): 73–38; Guinard, J., and Mazzucchelli, R. (1996). The sensory perception of texture and mouthfeel. *Trends in Food Science & Technology* 7(7): 213–19; Martins, Y., and Pliner, P. (2006). "Ugh! That's disgusting!": Identification of the characteristics of foods underlying rejections based on disgust. *Appetite* 46(1): 75–85.

2. Lundy, B., et al. (1998). Food texture preferences in infants versus toddlers. *Early Child Development and Care* 146(1): 69–85; Oram, N. (1994). Children's eating experiences could differ from those of adults. *Appetite* 22(3): 283–7.

3. Baxter, I.A., Jack, F.R., and Schröder, M. (1998). The use of repertory grid method to elicit perceptual data from primary school children. *Food Quality and Preference* 9(1): 73–38; Nicklaus, S., et al. (2005). A prospective study of food variety seeking in childhood, adolescence and early adult life. *Appetite* 44(3): 289–97; Perez-Rodrigo, C., and Aranceta, J. (2003). Nutrition education in schools: experiences and challenges. *European Journal of Clinical Nutrition* 57: S82–S85.

School-Age Children: Smart Strategies for Raising Food-Savvy Kids

1. Weber, K., Story, M., and Harnack, L. (2006). Internet food marketing strategies aimed at children and adolescents: A content analysis of food and beverage brand web sites. *Journal of the American Dietetic Association* 106(9): 1463.

2. American Academy of Pediatrics. (2011). Media use by children younger than 2 years old. *Pediatrics* 128(5): 1040–45; American Academy of Pediatrics. (2005). *Caring for Your Baby and Child, from Birth to Age 5*. Washington: AAP.

3. Harris, J.L., Brownell, K.D., and Bargh, J.A. (2009). The food marketing defense model: Integrating psychological research to protect youth and inform public policy. *Social Issues and Policy Review* 3(1): 211–71.

4. Faith, M.S., et al. (2012). Parent–child feeding strategies and their relationships to child eating and weight status. *Obesity Research* 12(11): 1711–22.

5. van Strien, T., and Bazelier, F.G. (2007). Perceived parental control of food intake is related to external, restrained and emotional eating in 7- to 12-year-old boys and girls. *Appetite* 49(3): 618–25; Rodin, J. (1981). Current status of the internal–external hypothesis for obesity. *American Psychologist* 36: 361–72; Birch, L.L., Fisher, J.O., Davison, K.K. (2003). Learning to overeat: Maternal use of restrictive feeding practices promote girls' eating in the absence of hunger. *American Journal of Clinical Nutrition* 78(2): 215–20; Carper, J.L., Fisher, J.O., and Birch, L.L. (2000). Young girl's emerging dietary restraint and disinhibition are related to parental control in child feeding. *Appetite* 35(2): 121–9; Birch, L.L., and Fisher, J.O. (1998). Development of eating behaviors among children and adolescents. *Pediatrics* 101(3): 539–49.

6. Ogden, J., Reynolds, R., and Smith, A. (2006). Expanding the concept of parental control: A role for overt and covert control in children's snacking behaviour? *Appetite* 47(1): 100–106.

7. Antonovsky, A. (1987). *Unraveling the Mystery of Health: How People Manage Stress and Stay Well*. San Francisco: Jossey-Bass; Antonovsky, A. (1993, March). The structure and properties of the sense of coherence scale. *Social Science and Medicine* 36: 725–33; Ray, C, Suominen, S., and Roos, E. (2009). The role of parents' sense of coherence in irregular meal pattern and food intake pattern of children aged 10–11 in Finland. *Journal of Epidemiology and Community Health* 63(12): 1005–9.

Acknowledgments

This book was a labor of love to which many people contributed.

For tolerating my sometimes weird, sometimes wonderful attempts in the kitchen, my warmest thanks to two dozen test families scattered around the world: Babette, Brandy, Celine, Claire, Françoise, Greg, Jacqueline, Jamie, Jennifer, Jessica, Jon, Kristine, Lori, Roberta, Martha, Meg, Mira, Sarah Jane, Sophie, Stacy, Teresa, Trevor, and Beth, and their families, and all the children and caregivers at the Alphabet Academy—the most dedicated taste testers I could ever have hoped for!

Martha Magor Webb wore many hats: agent, taste tester, supportive critic, and friend. It's been a joy to work with her. Thanks, too, to the entire team at the Anne McDermid Agency.

Designing and daydreaming about illustrations with artist Sarah Jane Wright was the perfect inspiration for writing. Thanks, Sarah Jane, for your willingness to brainstorm and your endless patience!

Kate Cassaday (HarperCollins Canada) and Cassie Jones (William Morrow in New York) were, once again, a delight to work with: savvy, creative, insightful, and kind. I'm grateful to them and their colleagues for the enthusiasm they showed for the process, from beginning to end.

Last but not least: to Sophie, Claire, and Philippe—for your patience and for your loving, honest criticism. Who else would have put up with some of my wackier kitchen experiments? If I ever doubted that "food is love," you've put those doubts happily to rest.

Index